T0004613

The 30-Minute

# PREDIABETES COOKBOOK

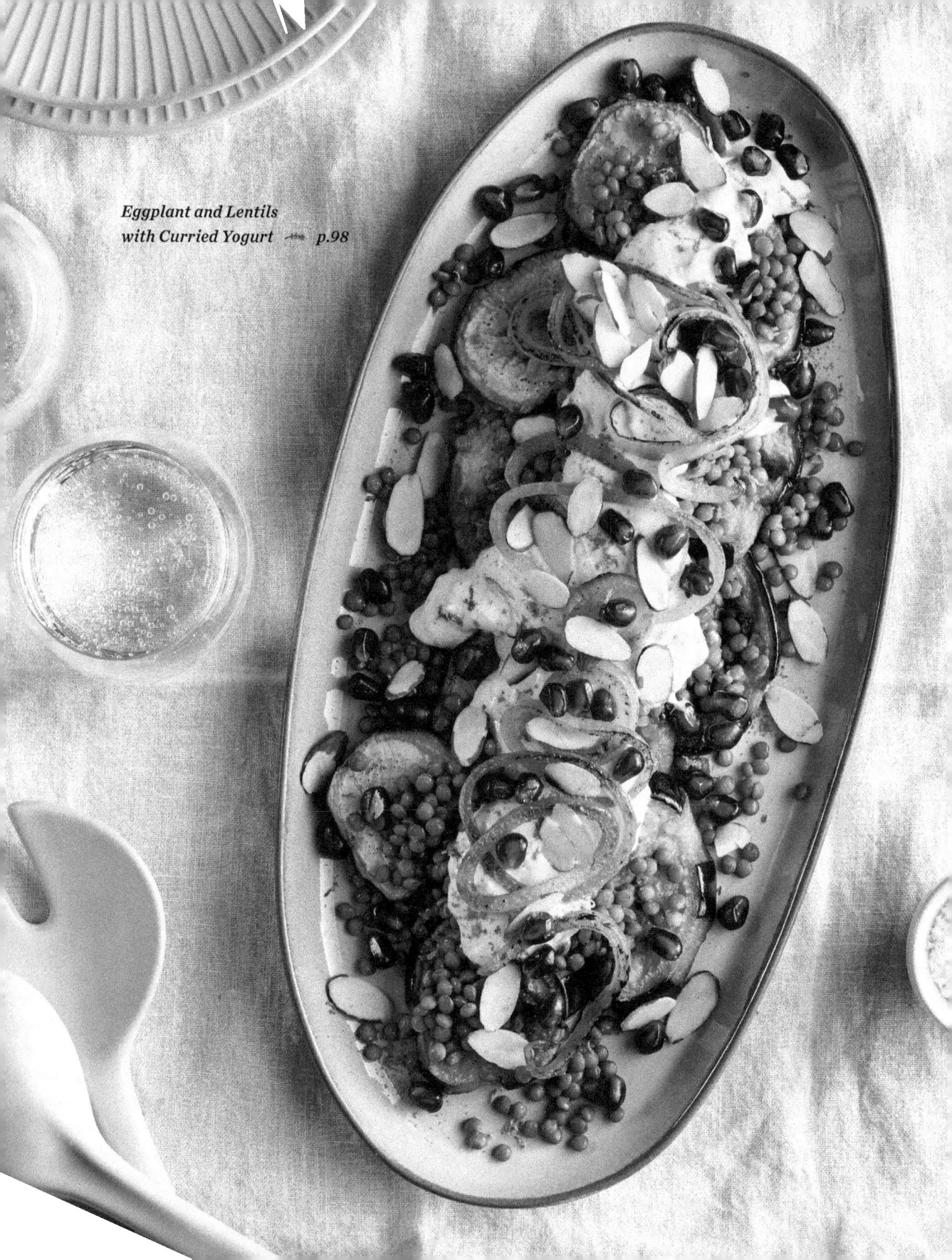

*Eggplant and Lentils with Curried Yogurt* p.98

# The 30-Minute PREDIABETES COOKBOOK

## 100 EASY RECIPES

to Improve and Manage Your Health through Diet

Photography by Elysa Weitala

Ranelle Kirchner, MS, RD, CDCES

ROCKRIDGE PRESS

*This book is dedicated to all of my patients and everyone in the fight for better health.*

Copyright © 2021 by Rockridge Press, Emeryville, California

No part of this publication may be reproduced, stored in a retrieval system, or transmitted in any form or by any means, electronic, mechanical, photocopying, recording, scanning, or otherwise, except as permitted under Sections 107 or 108 of the 1976 United States Copyright Act, without the prior written permission of the Publisher. Requests to the Publisher for permission should be addressed to the Permissions Department, Rockridge Press, 6005 Shellmound Street, Suite 175, Emeryville, CA 94608.

Limit of Liability/Disclaimer of Warranty: The Publisher and the author make no representations or warranties with respect to the accuracy or completeness of the contents of this work and specifically disclaim all warranties, including without limitation warranties of fitness for a particular purpose. No warranty may be created or extended by sales or promotional materials. The advice and strategies contained herein may not be suitable for every situation. This work is sold with the understanding that the Publisher is not engaged in rendering medical, legal, or other professional advice or services. If professional assistance is required, the services of a competent professional person should be sought. Neither the Publisher nor the author shall be liable for damages arising herefrom. The fact that an individual, organization, or website is referred to in this work as a citation and/or potential source of further information does not mean that the author or the Publisher endorses the information the individual, organization, or website may provide or recommendations they/it may make. Further, readers should be aware that websites listed in this work may have changed or disappeared between when this work was written and when it is read.

For general information on our other products and services or to obtain technical support, please contact our Customer Care Department within the United States at (866) 744-2665, or outside the United States at (510) 253-0500.

Rockridge Press publishes its books in a variety of electronic and print formats. Some content that appears in print may not be available in electronic books, and vice versa.

TRADEMARKS: Rockridge Press and the Rockridge Press logo are trademarks or registered trademarks of Callisto Media Inc. and/or its affiliates, in the United States and other countries, and may not be used without written permission. All other trademarks are the property of their respective owners. Rockridge Press is not associated with any product or vendor mentioned in this book.

Interior and Cover Designer: Monica Cheng
Art Producer: Sue Bischofberger
Editor: Anne Lowrey
Production Editor: Nora Milman

Photography © 2021 Elysa Weitala, with food styling by Victoria Woollard
Author photo courtesy of Chelsea Gortmaker

Cover: Roasted Tomato Tartine, page 73, and Minted Sweet Pea Soup, page 82

ISBN: Print 978-1-64739-324-3
eBook 978-1-64739-325-0
R1

# Contents

Introduction vii

CHAPTER ONE
Living with Prediabetes 1

CHAPTER TWO
Eating to Manage Your Prediabetes 15

CHAPTER THREE
Breakfast 31

CHAPTER FOUR
Salad 53

CHAPTER FIVE
Sandwiches and Soups 71

CHAPTER SIX
Mains 95

CHAPTER SEVEN
Sides and Snacks 123

CHAPTER EIGHT
Dessert 145

CHAPTER NINE
Seasonings, Sauces, and Dressings 157

Measurement Conversions 174

Resources 175

References 176

Index 179

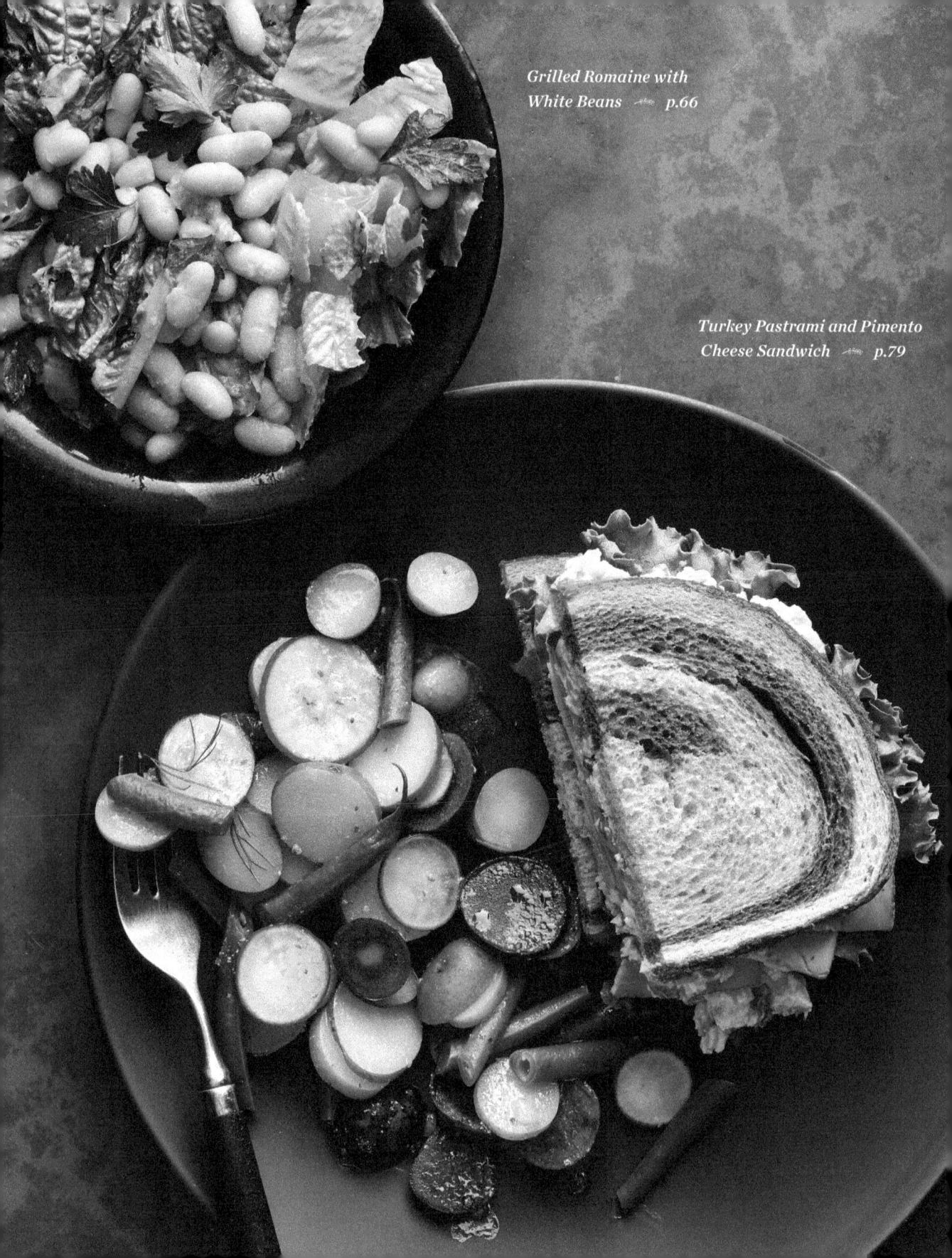

*Grilled Romaine with White Beans* p.66

*Turkey Pastrami and Pimento Cheese Sandwich* p.79

# Introduction

Congratulations! In opening this book, you've taken the all-important first step in achieving a healthier lifestyle and lowering your risk of diabetes. Every step counts, and it won't always be easy to make changes in your lifestyle. But rest assured, this book will be by your side to help make cooking a fun and simple piece in your health journey.

As a chef, registered dietitian, and certified diabetes educator, I understand the challenges people face when it comes to eating healthier. I also know, from personal experience, how difficult it is to change your diet. When I was a child, I loved "junk" food. Ice cream and French fries with ketchup were my favorites. I struggled with my weight and health for many years. Both sides of my family have a history of diabetes, heart disease, high cholesterol, hypertension, and more.

I started asking questions: Why am I overweight? Why do I feel this way? I want to feel better, but how do I make that happen? Once I understood the effect of food on the body, I made the gradual changes I needed. Lord knows it didn't happen overnight (and I'm still improving every day!). I now know I was not fueling my body with what it needed to function properly. Through my journey, I discovered my love of whole foods and cooking.

Cooking became my passion, and it flourished into a career. As I completed my internship at a Michelin-starred restaurant in Avignon, France, however, I knew I wanted to do more than cook. In France I developed a passionate interest in the relationship people have with the foods they eat. Upon returning home, I immediately enrolled at the University of Minnesota to become a registered dietitian. I wanted to show people how to improve their relationship with food by making simple, healthy changes. During this time I was cooking after class and on weekends, while saving every penny I could to take trips to more than 25 countries worldwide. Each has provided me great insight into various food cultures and traditions. This experience helped shape my recipes and the way I deliver care to people from all walks of life.

Although this book is designed to assist in preventing the onset of diabetes, the recipes and philosophies will apply to all types of diabetics, as well as anyone looking to maintain balance in their diet. The goal of this book is to introduce a variety of new foods and flavors to your palate while balancing carbohydrates and demonstrating how delicious "healthy" food can be. These recipes should spark excitement—because food *is* exciting—while also keeping the time spent in the kitchen to a minimum. Enjoy.

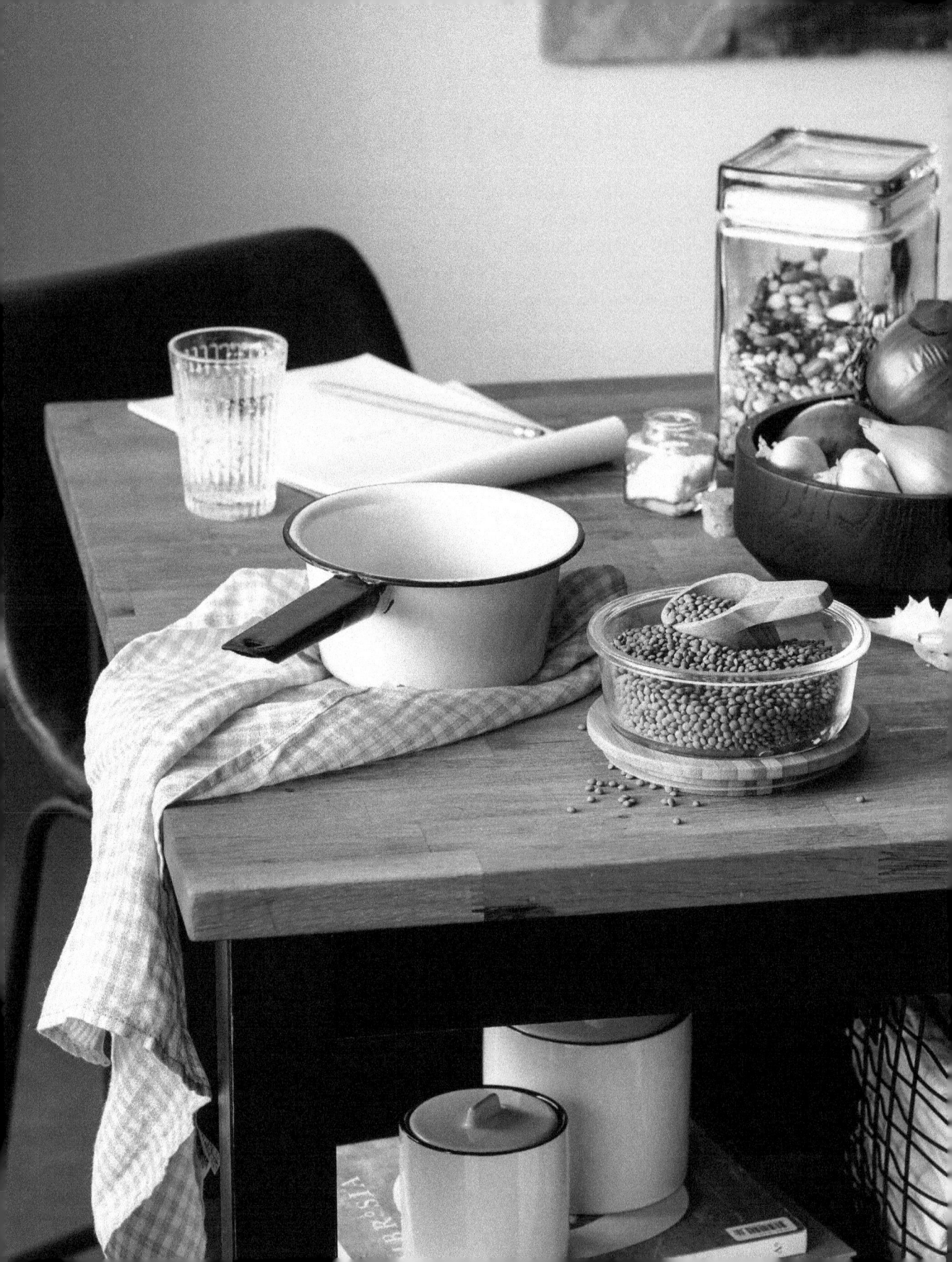

CHAPTER ONE

# Living with Prediabetes

Prediabetes is a serious global health concern. More than one in three American adults have prediabetes, and, according to the Centers for Disease Control and Prevention, up to 90 percent are unaware of their condition.

According to the American Diabetes Association, prediabetes may be reversible through the implementation of lifestyle changes, which include a healthier diet and increased exercise. It is challenging, however, to take the necessary steps while your busy schedule and the demands of daily life command so much time and attention. This time issue is the main reason I have limited the recipes to 30 minutes (or less): to help limit stress while maintaining nutritional balance.

In this chapter, you will learn more about prediabetes and how it differs from the diagnosis of diabetes. You will also become familiar with the current medical treatments of prediabetes through diet, medication, physical activity, and other ways to lower your risk in regard to developing into the next stage.

# Understanding Prediabetes

Prediabetes is a chronic metabolic condition that occurs when blood glucose levels rise higher than normal, but below the threshold for diabetes. Diagnosing prediabetes is based on laboratory values from more than one test and includes the following blood sugar measurements: fasting plasma glucose (FPG), impaired glucose tolerance (IGT—during the oral glucose tolerance test [OGTT]), and A1C or average blood glucose level. The IFG (impaired fasting glucose) and IGT show your blood glucose levels at the time you test your blood, and the A1C reflects your average blood glucose over the past 60 to 90 days.

| | Normal | Prediabetes | Diabetes |
|---|---|---|---|
| FPG | <100 mg/dL | 100–125 mg/dL | ≥126 mg/dL |
| IGT | <140 mg/dL | 140–199 mg/dL | ≥200 mg/dL |
| A1C | <5.7% | 5.7–6.4% | ≥6.5% |

Typically, prediabetes occurs in those who have some insulin resistance, which is when beta cells on the pancreas do not make enough insulin to keep blood glucose within a normal range. Insulin is an essential hormone in the body because without it, glucose stays in your blood and does not enter your cells. Think of insulin as a key. Glucose from the blood needs this key to unlock and enter the cell walls so that the cells can use the glucose as energy to deliver oxygen throughout your body.

## *The Causes of Prediabetes*

Prediabetes can be caused by various factors—many of which you cannot control. These uncontrollable factors are termed "non-modifiable risk factors." Other risk factors, however, you can regulate. Modifiable risk factors may require the use of medications, and others may take changing behaviors.

**Modifiable Risk Factors:**

- High blood pressure
- High levels of triglycerides
- Inactivity
- Low levels of high-density lipoprotein (HDL), the "good" cholesterol
- Excess weight or obesity
- Poor or inadequate diet

**Non-Modifiable Risk Factors:**

- Age 45 or older
- Ethnicity: Although it is unclear why, people of certain races—including African American, Alaska Native, South Asian, American Indian, Latino/Hispanic, Native Hawaiian, or Pacific Islander American—are more likely to develop prediabetes.
- Family history with type 2 diabetes from a parent, brother, or sister
- Gestational diabetes, which is diabetes during pregnancy, can affect both the mother and the child
- Personal history of heart disease or stroke
- Personal history of polycystic ovary syndrome (PCOS), a common condition characterized by irregular menstrual periods, excess hair growth, and obesity

**Also, there are risk factors that may contribute to insulin resistance; these include:**

- Cushing's syndrome, acromegaly, and other hormonal disorders
- Excess abdominal weight—the weight that accumulates around your midsection
- Medications like glucocorticoids, some types of HIV medications, and antipsychotics
- Obstructive sleep apnea or other sleep problems
- Tobacco smoke

If you are overweight or obese and have one or more of the other aforementioned risk factors for diabetes, you should be tested for prediabetes. If results are normal and you have other risk factors, you should retest at a minimum of every three years. The sooner you get tested, the sooner you can act to improve your health and, thus, the better your outcome will be in the long run.

## *How Prediabetes Can Affect You*

Blood sugar levels are often not high enough to cause chronic symptoms for most individuals. However, there is evidence that suggests some people with prediabetes may have early changes in their eyes, which can eventually lead to retinopathy. Retinopathy is damage to any part of the retina, which can cause blurry vision and permanent damage to your eyes. Blood vessels that lead to the eyes are microscopic, and when cells do not get the oxygen they need, the eyes become affected in many ways that can eventually lead to blindness.

In addition to the effect on the eyes, those who are prediabetic are at risk for developing type 2 diabetes. Even if you do not develop type 2 diabetes, prediabetes is also linked to cardiovascular disease and kidney damage because of the increased strain on the heart and demand on the kidneys.

Along with the effects on your body, prediabetes can also have major implications on your mental and emotional state. Sudden mood changes may occur, including nervousness, sadness, difficulty thinking, anger or anxiety, and feeling tired (low energy). These sudden changes and negative feelings are caused by an increase in blood sugar levels that influence emotional response and can cause emotional strain on all aspects of your personal life and relationships. A recent study from Wolf et al. at Iowa State University found that "People with type 2 diabetes and prediabetes were more likely to focus on and have a strong emotional response to threats and negative things, which affects quality of life and increases risk for depression."

While prediabetes is increasingly common, it's more important to note that it is reversible. This book can help anyone living with prediabetes (and diabetes) by aiding with the simple, proven lifestyle change known as "your diet."

# What to Know About the Types of Diabetes

Diabetes refers specifically to having high blood glucose. The causes of the higher levels of glucose varies, which is why there are different types of diabetes. The main and most talked-about types are type 1, type 2, and gestational diabetes (often abbreviated to GDM).

**Type 1 |** This form of diabetes is usually diagnosed in youth, but it can develop at any age and in people of every race, shape, and size. Type 1 diabetics either do not make insulin in their pancreas, or the insulin produced is not enough. This shortfall of insulin is caused by the immune system mistakenly attacking the cells that make insulin. It is less common than type 2 diabetes, and treatment options are limited to insulin injections. With nearly one-fifth of the population afraid of needles, this can be anxiety-inducing, especially when a child is told to take insulin injections for life. Carbohydrate counting is necessary, as well as understanding the effects of exercise and how to create a balance among these factors.

**Type 2 |** The most common form of diabetes is type 2. It's progressive and multifactorial. Insulin resistance and increased glucose production from the liver are hallmark features. When these factors are combined, more insulin is required to be released, but it cannot keep up with the high glucose levels. Over time, the cells that release the insulin cannot be maintained and lose their function, resulting in cell death and insulin deficiency. Heredity plays a key role in the presence of type 2 diabetes; however, it is the environmental influences that turn genes on or off. These are the previously discussed modifiable risk factors, including exposure to chemicals and medications.

**Gestational |** GDM is associated with insulin resistance due to pregnancy, possibly obesity, and genetics. It is also associated with an increased risk of diabetes for the mother after the birth. Maternal risks include cesarean delivery, hypertension, and polyhydramnios (an increase in amniotic fluid), which in turn increases the risk of morbidity and mortality. After delivery, blood sugars typically return to normal, but should continue to be checked 6 to 12 weeks postpartum.

## Current Treatments

The aforementioned diagnostic criteria from two laboratory values guide the treatment options available for people with diabetes. The landmark Diabetes Prevention Program (DPP) was a study on more than 14,000 high-risk people for prediabetes. This study demonstrated that interventions with intensive lifestyle modifications like improved eating, physical activity, and weight loss reduced incidence by 58 percent versus those who used medication intervention (metformin) that reduced their weight by 31 percent. A 10-year follow-up to the DPP study showed a reduction of diabetes by 34 percent in the lifestyle group versus 18 percent in the medication group.

More doctors are testing for prediabetes and diabetes with increased awareness, knowing the importance of early detection for immediate attention. Depending on the individual and their medical history, the treatment strategy should be tailored specifically to that person. Regardless of the treatment, it is well-advised for each individual, including family members and caretakers, to receive additional diabetes education. Consult a certified diabetes educator (CDE—recently changed to certified diabetes care and education specialist [CDCES]) and nutrition education from a registered dietitian.

### *Diet Modification*

Optimizing nutrition through a person's diet is the underlying principle of prediabetes lifestyle change recommendations. Choosing nutrient-dense, high-fiber foods in moderation instead of heavily processed foods with added sugar, fat, and sodium is a must. And let us not forget the addictive sugar-sweetened beverages that are a major culprit of increased blood sugars—cut soda out of your diet today. Every other type of food can be included in a healthy diet. It's about creating balance and choosing healthier foods such as lean protein sources and unsaturated fats, while drinking plenty of water and eating three to five servings of vegetables throughout the day.

When you start restricting food choices and using negative language when talking about food, it hurts your relationship with food. It is for this reason why this book uses ingredients that often get a bad rap, such as honey. When consumed in excess, honey can be harmful to your health, but when eaten in moderation within a balanced meal, honey can provide health benefits.

Another example is the ingestion of carbohydrates. It's a common myth that carbs are bad for you. They're not. Carbohydrates are the preferred source of fuel for the body, more specifically the brain and central nervous system. Some carbs are healthier than others, such as whole-grain, complex, and high-fiber foods. People view carbs negatively, but it's important not to forget the benefits they provide for your heart and that they keep you fuller longer (a double bonus!).

Creating a balance in macronutrients (carbohydrates, proteins, and fats) at each meal is fundamental, with an overall goal of weight loss using lifestyle modification. Think of weight loss as 80 percent eating and 20 percent exercise.

## *Medications*

Although lifestyle changes are the focus when it comes to prediabetes, medications may be recommended as well. Metformin therapy is most commonly prescribed and should be considered for prediabetics with body mass index (BMI) $\geq 35 kg/m^2$, those under 60 years of age, and women with prior GDM. Metformin improves blood glucose control by decreasing the amount of glucose the liver makes, decreasing the amount of glucose absorbed by the intestines, and improving insulin sensitivity.

People with prediabetes have a higher risk for cardiovascular disease (CVD). Prioritizing and treating CVD risk factors is crucial; therefore, equal emphasis must be given to hypertension and dyslipidemia. This is the reason why medications for these conditions may be warranted. A person's laboratory values, previous medical history, and anthropometrics such as waist circumference, weight, and BMI are used to determine treatment options and goals.

The number of cholesterol-lowering medications is vast. They are grouped into six drug classes, but the most recommended belong to statins, the only cholesterol-lowering drug class with a direct association in risk reduction of a heart attack or stroke.

You should have a 10-year risk assessment from your doctor to determine your need for cholesterol-lowering medications. They will weigh the pros and cons of medication therapy. Perhaps medications are not required and lifestyle changes alone may be all you need! This is why I am providing these easy, quick recipes to help with the diet component.

## *Embracing Exercise*

In addition to diet, it's essential to address your activity level when discussing risk reduction of prediabetes, diabetes, and living a healthier life. Recommendations are to get at least 150 minutes of exercise each week, or roughly 30 minutes at least five days a week.

Hopefully this doesn't send your jaw dropping to the floor, because this is only a suggestion. Everyone has their limitations, and it's always best to start slowly and gradually. If you don't exercise at all, this may seem impossible. The key is to choose something you love to do that gets your body moving. Maybe it's a brisk walk around the neighborhood, doing chair exercises in your home, or doing something completely new like snowshoeing. Bring a friend for support if that helps you stay on track.

You do not have to hit the gym and spend your money on expensive gym equipment or workout classes. Getting in a home workout is just as effective and can save you money. Using soup cans as weights or even your own body weight is a great place to start. Perhaps you start out doing 10 minutes of stretching in the morning and later in the day take a walk on your lunch break. Every minute counts!

In a society in which our time is of the essence, you may have the excuse of "There just isn't enough time to exercise and cook a nutritious meal." This book will give you the free time to put toward your workout. Many of the recipes can be made in advance or multiplied to save you even more precious time.

## Dietary Herbs and Supplements: Are They Worth It?

Nontraditional treatments consisting of dietary herbs and supplements are commonly used because these products often make promising claims. They do not require proof of safety, effectiveness, and purity, which is why you must be cautious and should consult with a registered dietitian and doctor before deciding to take supplements. Side effects and drug interactions are a high possibility.

Many of the products listed in the following chart have real effects that eventually may prove to be beneficial. However, at this point, these products lack the high-quality evidence of safety and effectiveness needed to recommend them for long-term use.

If supplements are something you take or are considering, make sure they are tested by a third party, like ConsumerLab.com, NSF International, or the US Pharmacopeia (USP). These organizations provide evaluations of supplements to help you decide which brands are reliable. They test the supplement ingredients for identity, strength, quality, and purity.

Above all, be sure to discuss the benefits and risks of any supplements or herbs with your doctor.

* These proposed recommendations are based solely on the Safety and Effectiveness Ratings contained in *Natural Medicines*.

Recommendation Chart for Natural Medicines Used for Diabetes

| EFFECTIVENESS | SAFETY | | | |
|---|---|---|---|---|
| | LIKELY SAFE | POSSIBLY SAFE | INSUFFICIENT EVIDENCE | POSSIBLY UNSAFE |
| LIKELY EFFECTIVE | | | | |
| POSSIBLY EFFECTIVE | American ginseng<br>Blond psyllium<br>Cassia cinnamon<br>Flaxseed<br>Magnesium<br>Oats<br>Soy<br>Xanthan gum | Aloe<br>Alpha-lipoic acid<br>Banaba<br>Chromium<br>Fenugreek<br>Glucomannan<br>Guarumo<br>Inulin<br>Ivy gourd<br>Prickly pear cactus<br>Siberian ginseng<br>White mulberry | | |
| INSUFFICIENT EVIDENCE | Coenzyme Q10<br>Stevia<br>Vanadium | Bitter melon<br>Chia<br>Gymnema<br>Asian ginseng<br>Common bean | | |
| POSSIBLY INEFFECTIVE | Flaxseed oil | | | Selenium |

Consider this product

Don't recommend using this product

Recommend against using this product

*Chart is modified from the Natural Medicines Database.*

### *Talk to Your Doctor*

Upon diagnosis, talk to your doctor to address any concerns you may have. They will guide you through key management strategies, answer your questions, and follow up with you on a regular basis to keep you on track to prevent diabetes from occurring. It is generally recommended to visit with your health provider at least every six months and more frequently if needed once diagnosed with prediabetes. As mentioned earlier, working with a certified diabetes educator and registered dietitian as well as your primary care provider can be instrumental in your journey to making lifestyle changes. They can help you stay on track with your health goals and provide counsel.

Consider asking these questions:

1. Why do I need to know about managing my blood sugars?
2. What are the symptoms of prediabetes?
3. What can I do to delay or prevent type 2 diabetes?
4. What are my risk factors for developing type 2 diabetes?
5. Are there support groups I can attend?
6. What lifestyle changes can I make to reduce my risk of prediabetes or diabetes?
7. What, if any, medications would you recommend I take to prevent type 2 diabetes, including those related to blood pressure and cholesterol?
8. Is there a National Diabetes Prevention Program organization I can join that's local?
9. How is my diet influencing my blood sugars?

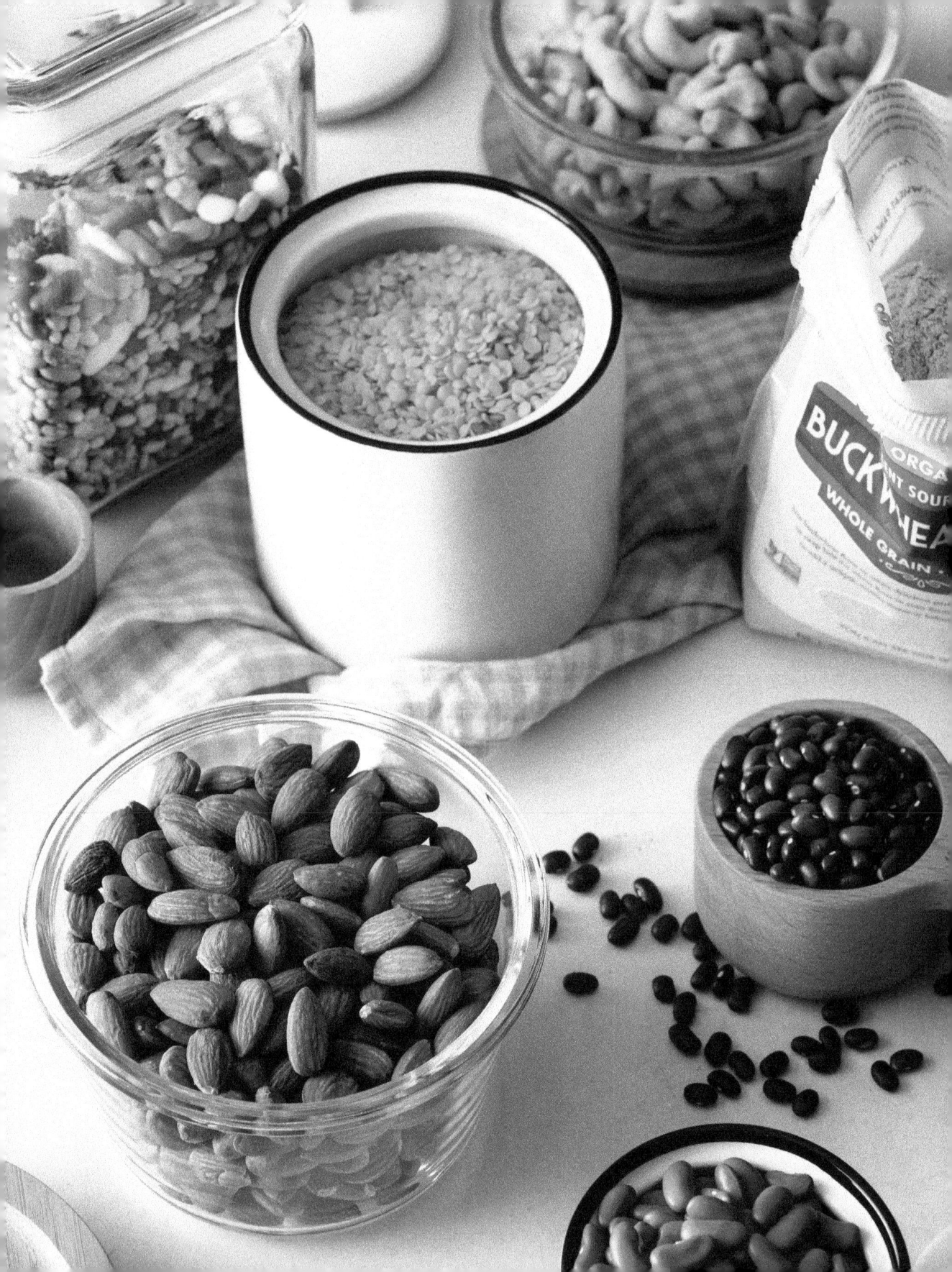
BUCKWHEA
ORGA
NT SOUR
WHOLE GRAIN

CHAPTER TWO

# Eating to Manage Your Prediabetes

What you feed your body affects all aspects of your health, as well as your current and future state of being. It's important to remember that you may not be able to tell if someone is healthy only by looking at them—people come in all shapes and sizes. The decisions you make about what you eat can have extreme consequences for your body over time, especially if you have prediabetes or a chronic disease like diabetes. Read on to learn more and to understand how your diet specifically affects your health and well-being.

## The Link between Food and Prediabetes

Your diet plays an incredibly important role in regulating health and wellness, affecting the potential for developing significant diseases like diabetes. Food is made up of protein, fat, and carbohydrates and acts as fuel for the body, keeping it functioning properly. While you may not always see how food affects the body, at a metabolic level the foods you choose to eat impact everything from stress to sleep to energy levels and mood.

The key source of fuel for your body comes from the carbohydrates found in food. These are separated into three main groups: starch, sugar, and fiber. Carbs are not popular in many diets lately, but they remain essential to your health. Some are healthier than others, as they take longer to process in the body and keep you full for longer: Whole-grains, whole fruits, beans, and vegetables are all excellent sources of carbohydrates. Less desirable are simpler carbs, which get used for energy quickly—these include white bread, white rice, juice, soda, and candy. When we consume these simple carbohydrate foods in excess, our bodies have difficulty naturally controlling our blood sugars. Foods with starch and sugar get broken down into glucose, but over time an excess of glucose builds in our blood, and that can lead to prediabetes and diabetes. Couple this with inadequate sleep and water consumption, increased stress, poor diet, and a lack of exercise (among other risk factors), and the risk for diabetes increases.

## *Sugar and the Glycemic Index*

Sugar is one of the main types of carbohydrates found in foods, which provide your body with energy. Let's take it even further to distinguish between naturally occurring sugars and added sugars. The sugars found in milk and fruit are naturally occurring examples. The sugar found in processed foods, like the syrup in canned fruit or baked goods like cookies, was added during preparation. Foods with added sugars have a higher impact on your blood sugars, as they are processed much more quickly in the body.

The best ways to watch sugar levels include:

- serving yourself smaller portions and making your own food at home
- avoiding "flavored" products such as strawberry yogurt (add fresh strawberries to plain yogurt instead)
- swapping out soda for water
- eating more protein and fat
- checking food labels for sugar amounts, as packaging can sometimes be misleading
- focusing on whole foods with no sugar added

A glycemic index (GI) is used to help understand the impact of food on blood sugar. More specifically, a GI provides a value for foods, which gives us an idea of exactly *how* quickly (or slowly) these foods cause your blood sugar levels to increase. Foods with a lower GI, such as beans and milk, tend to release glucose slowly and steadily, while higher GI foods, such as potatoes, white bread, and white rice, release glucose rapidly.

The reason GI can be a beneficial tool for those with prediabetes and diabetes is that it acts as a guide for healthy decision-making. The GI is not the only benchmark to use when considering food; the total amount of carbohydrates and overall nutritional quality is important as well. Those with prediabetes or diabetes, or at risk, can choose foods with a lower GI to nurture weight loss and provide better blood glucose control. On the other hand, high GI foods play an important role in energy recovery after a workout and can help offset low blood sugars.

## *Understanding Carbohydrates*

A common myth about those with prediabetes or diabetes is that they must avoid carbohydrates. The fact remains, carbohydrates are essential to the body, providing the bulk of its fuel. Rather than avoiding carbohydrates, the key is to understand how to eat them in moderation to keep blood sugars in check, while focusing on eating more of the healthier types of carbohydrates.

Another way to think about carbohydrates is based on their chemical structure, notably those that are simple (sometimes called simple sugars) or complex (starch). The most significant difference between the two is how quickly the body digests and absorbs each.

Simple carbohydrates are found in natural foods like fruit, milk, and some vegetables, but they are also found in many processed foods. These types of carbohydrates break down rather quickly and, when eaten in excess, can spike blood sugars.

Structurally, complex carbohydrates are made up of long chains of sugars that require a longer time for the body to break down. Whole-grain foods and starchy vegetables are the bulk of these foods, but there are also refined starches that are technically complex, such as cakes, pastries, and white bread. When dietitians advise "eating more complex," they are referring to whole-grain foods and starchy vegetables because of their slower absorption, keeping you fuller for longer. Refined carbohydrates lack the fiber that is found in whole grains because of the processing the food undergoes. In fact, refined carbs can sometimes raise blood glucose levels as quickly as simple sugars.

## *Cholesterol, the Good (and the Bad) Kind*

Cholesterol is an essential waxy substance found in many foods and within our cells. It is used to make hormones and vitamin D and in the digestive process. Two main types of cholesterol, the "good" and the "bad," seem to be mentioned frequently, but there is also another primary type called very low-density lipoprotein (VLDL) that promotes plaque buildup.

How do you know which cholesterol is good or bad?

"Good" refers to high-density lipoprotein or HDL. Think of the "H" as a helper, because it helps remove excess cholesterol in your blood and transport it back to your liver, where it is broken down and removed from the body. Examples of foods that help increase your HDL are whole grains and plants with high fiber, fish, and plant-based fats such as extra-virgin olive oil, avocado, flax, and chia seeds.

"Bad" refers to low-density lipoprotein or LDL. You can remember this by associating the "L" with the word "lousy." LDL can lead to a buildup of plaque in the arteries and narrowing of the passageways. Sometimes a clot can develop and get stuck, causing a heart attack or stroke. It is for these reasons that you should limit the foods that increase your LDL cholesterol: beef, lamb, poultry, pork, butter, cream, coconut, and palm oil.

## The Seven Self-Care Behaviors

Diabetes care and education specialists developed seven key areas for those diagnosed with prediabetes or diabetes. The ADCES (Association of Diabetes Care & Education Specialists) uses a framework called the "Seven Self-Care Behaviors." These behaviors are essential for successful and effective diabetes self-management outcomes.

1. **Healthy eating:** Having diabetes doesn't mean you can't enjoy the foods you love, but you need to know how food affects your blood sugars. Learn how your current diet affects your health and which gradual changes to make for positive impact.

2. **Being active:** It's not only about weight loss. Being active can help lower cholesterol, improve blood pressure, lower stress/anxiety, lower blood sugars, and improve your mood.

3. **Monitoring:** When you test your blood sugars at different times, before and after activity, and before and after eating, you will see how your lifestyle affects your blood sugars. Regular checks mean you can take action sooner and improve your sugars faster.

4. **Taking medication:** It's essential to take your medications as prescribed and know how they work. There are several that are often recommended and required due to the complexity of managing health during diabetes.

5. **Problem solving:** Learning how to problem-solve is important for managing prediabetes and diabetes. There's no one-size-fits-all approach to diabetes, so it's important to figure out what works best for you.

6. **Healthy coping:** Both your emotions and body can be affected by diabetes; it's natural. Coping means taking steps to lower the negative impact your emotions may have on your self-care.

7. **Reducing risks:** Having diabetes puts you at a higher risk of developing other serious health conditions. It's important to know what they are and how you can reduce them.

## A New Approach to Food

Food is exciting, and I'm going to prove that with the recipes in this book. I challenge you to try something new and look at food differently. You don't have to make dramatic changes to your diet and avoid the foods you love. It's all about moderation and fitting in the foods you love with a focus on plant-based choices. There are countless culinary variations in this book that you likely haven't tried or eaten before now. That can be intimidating if you are in a food rut.

How do I recommend breaking out of that rut? Start with one new food. Cook it several different ways: roast, sauté, bake, stuff, steam, and more. You'll likely enjoy eating the new food in one of these preparations. If you try something 8 to 10 times, odds are you will grow to like it. How amazing! You can train your palate to enjoy nutritious foods, but you don't have to do it alone. The entire family can benefit, so do this together. Your heart, mind, body, and spirit will thank you for it.

### *Foods to Embrace*

Eat to feel good by making sure you are getting plenty of whole fruits, vegetables, and grains; lean meats; plant-based protein, like unsalted nuts and seeds; and less added sugar and processed foods. You may recognize that some of these foods contain carbohydrates—these are the healthier sources. They should not be avoided.

Common diabetes superfoods are those rich in vitamins, minerals, antioxidants, and fiber, including:

**Beans** are high in fiber, magnesium, and potassium.

**Berries** are packed with antioxidants, vitamins such as vitamin K and C, manganese, potassium, and fiber. They are perfect for those sweet cravings you may encounter.

**Dairy products** like milk and yogurt are rich in vitamin D and calcium. Look for plain yogurt instead of flavored, and if you want more bang for your nutrition buck, try Greek yogurt.

**Dark green, leafy vegetables,** such as spinach, collards, kale, and chard, are packed with iron, calcium, and potassium, and vitamins A, C, E, and K.

**Omega-3 fatty acids** from fish, nuts, and seeds are healthy fats that help keep you fuller longer.

**Plant-based milk** is a wonderful alternative to dairy if you are trying to cut down on carbohydrates at a meal. They are easy to make but are also widely available at many stores. If you can, look for unsweetened versions.

**Sweet potatoes, yams, and colored potatoes** are high in antioxidants, vitamins, and fiber. They are more nutritious than white potatoes.

**Whole grains** are rich in magnesium, B vitamins, chromium, iron, folate, and fiber. Some of the heavy hitters in this category include farro, millet, quinoa, barley, and oats.

## *Foods to Eat in Moderation*

These are the foods you need to approach with caution and eat less frequently, but remember, you don't have to avoid them entirely. An excess of the following foods and ingredients contributes to weight gain, increased blood sugar, and increase in the risk of heart disease. Although these foods get a bad rap, they are still food, and food is fuel. The reason these foods should be consumed less often is that they offer little nutritional value, are high in calories, may spike your blood sugar, or pose a health risk when eaten in abundance.

Eat less:

**Saturated fats.** Animal proteins, palm oil, coconut, and junk foods like chips, fried foods, and sweets contain these less-healthy fats.

**Trans fats.** Junk foods as well as packaged foods, margarine, frozen meals, muffins, and other baked goods contain trans fats because they lengthen the shelf life of food. Trans fats are linked to insulin resistance, heart disease, inflammation, and weight gain.

**Cholesterol.** High-cholesterol foods impact your heart. Keep red meats (such as beef, lamb, and pork) and some seafood (such as shrimp) to a minimum and consume lean meats. Eggs are an excellent source of protein, but the yolks contain nearly half your daily quota of cholesterol.

**Sodium.** High-sodium foods like deli meats, pickles, sauces, and condiments can increase your blood pressure and risk of hypertension.

**Sugar-sweetened cereals.** These increase your chances of high blood sugars.

**Refined foods.** White bread and white pasta are stripped of their original fiber, so they process much faster in the body and can spike our blood sugars.

### *When to Eat and How Often*

Timing is everything, especially if you are taking medications to help manage your blood sugar. Eating around the same time, with four to six hours between larger meals, is highly recommended because your body can regulate your blood sugars more efficiently. Data suggest that making changes to promote more regular intake of energy during the day has positive effects on risk factors for heart disease and diabetes.

Breakfast should be the first meal of the day and never skipped. Eating within one to two hours of waking up will provide your body with the energy it needs to work more efficiently. When breakfast intake decreases, obesity and chronic disease increase. Several studies have proven this association, which is why eating breakfast is recommended as a strategy to reach a healthy body weight. Additionally, studies report negative side effects for those who skip breakfast. Their blood sugars remained high even after other meals in the day, they felt hungrier, and they typically ate more at the end of the day.

Although it can be tempting to snack late at night before bedtime, many studies would suggest you rethink eating that cookie. Late-night eating increased the risk of obesity and, combined with skipping breakfast, showed an increase in metabolic syndrome in a study of 60,800 people, ages 20 through 75. Metabolic syndrome is characterized by high blood pressure, high blood sugar, excess fat around the midline, and abnormal cholesterol levels.

## Portioning Plates

Perhaps you've heard of MyPlate, the USDA's initiative that defines a healthy plate. It's an excellent place to start when thinking of how you could create balanced meals without having to crunch numbers and measure all your food. You're going to love how simple this tool is, because many Americans already eat in this fashion.

First of all, think of a 9-inch plate, not a 12-inch plate. Then divide your plate in half. This is your recommended nonstarchy vegetable portion, like leafy greens, tomatoes, eggplant, carrots, beets, onions, Brussels sprouts, cauliflower, peppers, or cucumber. What remains are two quarters of the plate. One quarter is designated as the protein portion, including meats, cheese, tofu, or fish. Think about a deck of cards; this is a proper serving of protein at each meal. The remaining quarter is for starchy, carbohydrate foods such as whole grains and starchy vegetables like beans, peas, tubers, and potatoes. Lastly, beyond the well-organized plate, you can have a side serving of fruit, milk, or plant-based milk. It's truly that easy.

Not every meal you choose to eat will follow this system, but at least it's a good place to start so you don't feel overwhelmed. Eating can be challenging, so do what's most comfortable for you. If this simple system helps, then, by all means, use it.

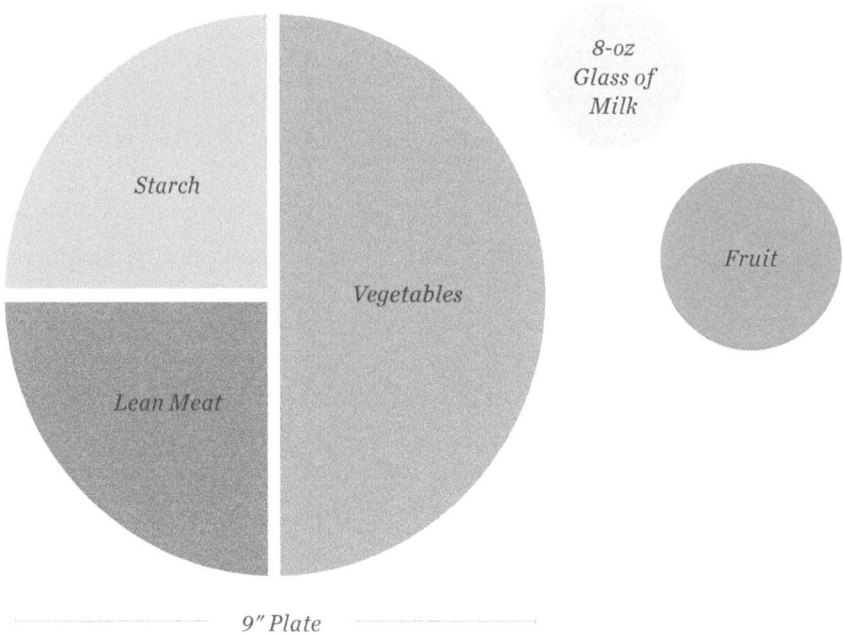


## Setting Up Your Kitchen

Now let's take a moment to think about your kitchen so you can set yourself up for success. If you don't have the tools or space to create healthy meals, meal prep becomes challenging, so consider your kitchen setup. Is it a clean, welcoming space with room to prepare your foods? Clear your kitchen of mail, keys, clothes, and anything else that doesn't belong. Organization ensures your time in the kitchen is productive, safe, and fun! Countertops and surfaces used for cooking should be kept clean at all times. The easiest way to keep your kitchen fresh and tidy is to clean as you go. Wipe up spills as they occur and while you are cooking. There's typically a pause in most recipes, so use that time to put ingredients away in the pantry or wash dirty dishes.

Another critical element when setting up your kitchen is to make sure it is well stocked with food and equipment. This doesn't mean packing the space with products, it means having some essentials on hand and planning out your week of meals ahead of time when you can. If you run low on an ingredient or need a piece of equipment, write it down to remind yourself to purchase it the next time you go to the store. Before you start cooking, be sure to read through recipes in their entirety. It would be a bummer to have to run all the way back to the store after you've started cooking.

## *Foods to Stock*

The most important part of your kitchen is the foods you stock. This means having a variety of ingredients that inspire you to cook and that you enjoy eating. These choices should store well in the freezer or pantry and allow you to make fast-and-easy meals. The bulk of these items should have a relatively long shelf life as well. Here's what I recommend.

### REFRIGERATOR

- Cheese
- Citrus, such as lime, lemon, or orange
- Eggs
- Favorite sauces and condiments
- Fresh herbs
- Milk or plant-based milk
- Plain yogurt
- Variety of fresh produce

### FREEZER

- Frozen vegetables
- Homemade broth and sauces
- Leftovers
- Protein (raw or cooked), including previously cooked beans and grains

### PANTRY

*Spices*

- Black pepper
- Cayenne pepper
- Chili powder
- Cinnamon
- Cloves
- Cumin
- Dried herbs, such as rosemary, oregano, thyme, and bay leaves
- Fennel seeds
- Ground coriander
- Kosher salt

- Paprika
- Red pepper flakes
- Spice blends, such as Italian seasoning mix, taco seasoning, and curry powder
- Turmeric

*Vegetables*

- Garlic
- Onions
- Sweet potatoes

*Oils and Vinegars*

- Cider vinegar
- Extra-virgin olive oil
- Grapeseed or canola oil
- Red wine vinegar

*Preserved Ingredients—low or no sodium added*

- Canned cooked beans and lentils
- Canned tomatoes
- Canned tomato paste
- Canned tuna, fish, and chicken
- Canned vegetables

*Starches*

- Couscous
- Noodles, such as rice noodles, buckwheat, and macaroni
- Variety of dried beans and lentils
- Variety of whole grains, such as rice, bulgur, quinoa, and oats

*Sauces and Condiments*

- Broth
- Dijon mustard
- Honey
- Pasta sauce
- Salad dressings
- Salsa
- Tamari or soy sauce
- Unsweetened, unsalted peanut butter (or other nut butter)

*Nuts and Seeds*

- Almonds
- Chia seeds
- Flaxseed
- Peanuts
- Seeds, such as pumpkin, sesame, and sunflower
- Walnuts

*Other Essentials*

- Baking powder
- Baking soda
- Bouillon cubes, low-sodium
- Cocoa powder, unsweetened
- Coconut, shredded and unsweetened
- Dried fruits
- Lemon juice
- Powdered milk
- Tofu (refrigerated or shelf-stable)

## *Essential Equipment*

Having gadgets and tools makes life more comfortable in the kitchen, but there is a point at which you can have too many. It can get expensive, and if you have limited storage space, that's also an issue. Here is a list of suggested equipment for your prediabetic kitchen, and keep in mind that if it's electronic, you can always do it the old fashioned way: by hand.

### KITCHEN ESSENTIALS

- Baking sheets: two or three, and ideally identical, so they are easy to stack and store
- Blender
- Box grater: Can be used for zesting and shredding cheese and vegetables.
- Casserole dish or Dutch oven: Heatproof cookware is great to have, especially if it has a lid.
- Colander: Make sure the holes aren't too small if you want to double it up for rinsing grains, pasta, berries, or produce. Otherwise, get one with larger holes and another one with smaller holes.
- Cutting board: One large and one small will do the trick.
- Flat spatula: Use with nonstick pans.
- Kitchen shears
- Measuring cups and spoons: Accuracy is often crucial for recipe success, especially in baking.
- Mixing bowls: A combination of sizes that nest inside one another makes for better storage.

- Nonstick frying pan
- Pastry brush
- Saucepan: I recommend a 4-quart saucepan, the size commonly used for making sauces.
- Sharp knives: You don't need more than a chef's knife and a paring knife. Keep them sharp, too; a dull knife is more dangerous than a sharp one.
- Skillet: One medium to large in size, with a lid, will allow you to prepare many foods on the stove top.
- Stockpot: Get one with a fitted lid that's easy to lift.
- Thermometer: Use for meats to verify doneness.
- Vegetable peeler
- Whisk
- Wooden spoons

### KITCHEN EXTRAS TO MAKE COOKING FASTER AND EASIER

- Bread knife: This blade is designed to cut bread but is also perfect for slicing through wraps, sandwiches, and tomatoes.
- Citrus juicer or reamer: This will make it easier to squeeze fresh citrus juice.
- Food processor: This appliance will save you boatloads of time on bean dips, doughs, and preparing vegetables.
- Immersion (hand-held) blender: This tool can be purchased with many attachments that allow you to whisk, process food in place of a food processor, and puree your foods. It's a great all-in-one electronic gadget.
- Mandoline: Allows you to get even, consistent slices every time.
- Microplane: This tool is for zesting citrus and grating hard cheeses, nutmeg, fresh ginger, and garlic cloves.
- Pressure cooker: Shortens the cooking time of whole grains, beans, stews, and meats.
- Salad spinner: Cleans your greens without using paper towels or cloth to dry them.

### *Where to Grocery Shop*

Not sure where to shop for some of the pantry staples? Try your local co-ops, grocery stores, farmers' markets, and international markets. The latter are generally family-run and not chains, which means you'll have to look them up online or ask around. You might be surprised by the ingredients found in these smaller stores. Typically, in larger US cities there is at least one market specializing in cuisines such as East Asian, Korean, African, Hispanic, or Indian. The food prices are generally lower, and you're supporting your local economy, so it's a win-win for the store and you. If you stick to larger grocery stores, visit the bulk-bin aisle to see what is available. Bulk items are often cheaper, and they allow you to experiment with new foods without committing to an entire bag of something you may not enjoy eating. Bring your own bags, containers, or glass jars to fill up in these sections. It's better for the environment, and it's nice to make sure sustainability is considered in your food purchases.

## About the Recipes

Every recipe in this book will take 30 minutes or less from start to finish. In addition to time, much consideration was put toward variety, ease, plant-based foods, and availability of ingredients while emphasizing cross-culture recipes. It's how I eat and how I encourage others to eat. Some ingredients may seem exotic to you, like bison, but I'll guide you on alternatives while also challenging your taste buds to try something new. Don't let the names of foods or recipes fool you either. Don't ignore a recipe just because a title may include a word or food you are unfamiliar with; instead, use it as an opportunity to learn and expand your repertoire with new flavors. There are thousands of different foods available, and this book is meant to open your eyes to the possibilities.

Substitution recommendations are also offered, so you don't feel glued to a recipe. One of the most common things I hear about from patients is how stuck they feel when it comes to recipes. If one ingredient is missing, they throw their hands in the air and say, "Forget it, I can't do this!" I'm going to challenge you to look beyond the recipe, use my tips to make adjustments, and use the recipe as a guideline. Just like it takes time to make changes to your lifestyle, it is a process to become comfortable in the kitchen.

Lastly, feel free to adjust the salt and pepper in most of the recipes. You will decide if you want to omit the seasonings or add salt and pepper to taste. The idea behind this is to try the recipe as is and keep your sodium intake lower. But food should be enjoyable, and some recipes may need a pinch of salt or dash of black pepper to perk them up. I am confident you will love the recipes in this book—just as my patients have for years.

## *How They're Easy*

The recipes in this book are meant to be quick, with little prep, to avoid having to stand for long periods in the kitchen. Most people do not want to spend their free time preparing food. I understand that spending more than 30 minutes on one meal is not compatible with a busy schedule. Extensive kitchen time is also not always possible for people who suffer from physical limitations.

These recipes are fast, easy, and use minimal kitchen equipment. You don't need a bunch of gadgets to make quick, healthy meals. Ingredients in this book should be easy to find at your local grocer. The recipes in this book also promote variety in your diet, so you can experience different flavors and ingredients with minimal effort and fuss.

## *Carb Counts and Nutritional Information*

Looking at the nutritional information provided for the recipes is helpful if you know how to interpret it. Always take into account your portion size and multiply or divide if you do not eat the recommended serving. For example, if you consume an entire smoothie in a recipe and it is two servings, you need to multiply the data by two. The nutrition information you see listed is what you would find on an FDA nutrition label, which explains where the calories are coming from (carbohydrate, protein, and fat), then a further breaks down the common nutrients, vitamins, and minerals that are of concern in a standard American diet. As a prediabetic or diabetic, the primary macronutrient of concern is total carbohydrates. Work with a dietitian or CDCES to determine how many servings or total carbohydrates are appropriate for you.

In most cases, adults should not exceed 75 grams of carbohydrates per meal. It is more commonly recommended to have between three to five servings per meal, so 45 to 75 grams per meal. As we discussed, there are many types of carbohydrates, but all will affect your blood sugars. Fiber will have more of a stabilizing effect on your blood sugars, and any recipe containing more than 5 grams per serving is considered to be a "good source" of fiber.

## *Recipe Labels and Tips*

All the recipes will be 30 minutes or less, with prep included. Amazing, right? Not only will you be guaranteed less time in the kitchen than your typical recipes, but there will be labels to help guide your decision to make it easy, too. Simply look for the following:

**5-Ingredient:** Recipes are made with five or fewer ingredients.

**Gluten-Free:** No gluten in the recipe; however, you'll want to read through the list of store-bought ingredients to make sure you have a gluten-free version. Tamari, Worcestershire sauce, miso, and certain grains like oats sometimes contain or come in contact with gluten.

**High-Fiber:** Contains 5 grams or more fiber per serving, which is great for keeping your blood sugars stabilized and keeping you fuller longer.

**No-Cook:** No heat necessary for these recipes. Simply chop, toss, and serve.

**One Pot, One Pan, One Bowl:** One and done, because it's nice to keep your cleanup to one thing.

**Vegetarian:** No meat, but can contain dairy, cheese, honey, or eggs. You'll find that many of these recipes are vegan, or easily made vegan, as well.

Look for these labels to help you see beyond the recipes and get creative, or to simply give you more information.

**Ingredient Tip:** How to best work with a particular ingredient.

**Make It Easier:** Shortcuts or kitchen tricks to make your cooking process even easier.

**Nutrient Boost:** My suggestions for adding extra nutrients to a recipe.

**Substitution Tip:** When and how you can substitute an ingredient for another.

**Variation:** Small recipe or ingredient changes for varying a recipe.

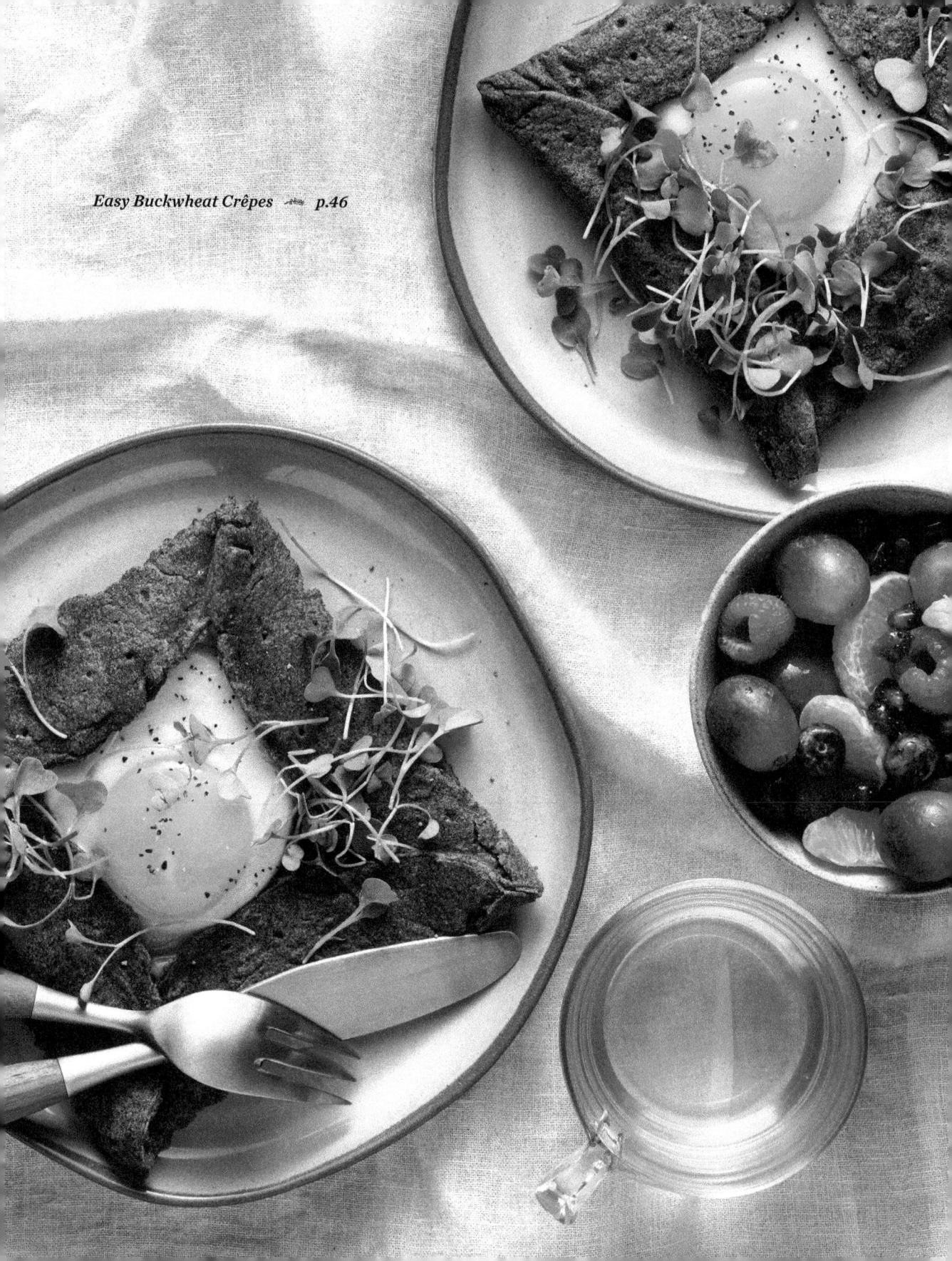

*Easy Buckwheat Crêpes* p.46

CHAPTER THREE

# Breakfast

Your morning meal becomes much easier and more enjoyable with these 16 reliable recipes. Most of the recipes in this chapter take less than 15 minutes to prepare, and you may be surprised to see that many include vegetables. Getting three to five servings of vegetables a day is challenging, but these recipes will help you integrate vegetables early in the day.

Breakfast foods are typically high in carbohydrates, and it can be hard to create a balance that keeps carbs in check. It's not that you *can't* eat them, but rather *how many* you consume in one meal. Think whole grains, and pair them with foods that do not spike your blood sugars, such as protein, nonstarchy vegetables, and fat, and you're on your way to a strong start to the day.

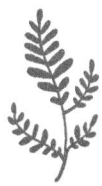

Blueberry-Chia Smoothie ..... 33

Cherry, Chocolate, and Almond Shake ..... 34

Stovetop Granola ..... 35

Seedy Muesli ..... 37

Overnight Oats ..... 38

Apple Millet Porridge ..... 40

Breakfast Banana Barley ..... 41

Harvest Blackberry Quinoa Bowl ..... 42

High-Protein Oatmeal ..... 43

Carrot Cake Oatmeal ..... 44

Strawberry-Ricotta Toast ..... 45

Easy Buckwheat Crêpes ..... 46

Shakshuka ..... 47

Eggplant Breakfast Sandwich ..... 48

Perfect Egg Scramble with Simple Salad ..... 49

Avocado-Tofu Scramble with Roasted Potatoes ..... 50

# Blueberry-Chia Smoothie

*Serves 2 / Prep time: 5 minutes*

**5-INGREDIENT, GLUTEN-FREE, HIGH-FIBER, NO-COOK, ONE POT, VEGETARIAN**

The blueberries in this delicious smoothie are a good source of vitamin C, an essential vitamin that also promotes wound healing. They are also high in fiber and manganese, which help the body better process cholesterol and carbohydrates. Couple that with chia seeds, a superfood high in omega fats and fiber, and you have a rich, fruity drink that is ideal for jump-starting your day.

**2 cups frozen blueberries**
**½ medium frozen banana**
**2 tablespoons peanut butter**
**2 tablespoons chia seeds**
**12 ounces unsweetened soy milk, plus extra if needed**

1. Combine the blueberries, banana, peanut butter, chia seeds, and soy milk in a blender and blend on high speed until smooth. Use a spatula to scrape down the sides as needed.
2. Serve immediately. If it's too thick, add more soy milk or water by the tablespoonful until you've reached the desired consistency.

**VARIATION:** Don't have blueberries on hand? Substitute any frozen berry, like strawberries or raspberries. Buy them in bulk when in season or on sale and freeze for later use. It will save you money in the long run, if you have the freezer space.

**INGREDIENT TIP:** I like to use ground chia seeds for this recipe for a smoother consistency. Simply grind them into a powder with a mini coffee grinder or mortar and pestle before using.

**Per serving:** Calories: 360; Total fat: 16g; Carbohydrates: 46g; Fiber: 14g; Protein: 12g; Calcium: 333mg; Vitamin D: 2mcg; Vitamin $B_{12}$: 2mcg; Iron: 2mg; Zinc: 1mg

# Cherry, Chocolate, and Almond Shake

*Serves 2 / Prep time: 5 minutes*

**5-INGREDIENT, GLUTEN-FREE, HIGH-FIBER, NO-COOK, ONE POT, VEGETARIAN**

The combination of cherry, chocolate, and almond is perfect culinary harmony. Cherries have floral, spicy flavor notes, and their pits share a common flavor with almonds. This synchronicity makes the two ingredients sing together in unison. In fact, the molecule that is produced from both of these foods, called benzaldehyde, is the second most commonly used flavor molecule in the United States after vanillin. Adding the cocoa simply enhances a winning combination, balancing the sweetness with a hint of bitterness.

**10 ounces frozen cherries**
**2 tablespoons cocoa powder**
**2 tablespoons almond butter**
**2 tablespoons hemp seeds**
**8 ounces unsweetened almond milk**

Combine the cherries, cocoa, almond butter, hemp seeds, and almond milk in a blender and blend on high speed until smooth. Use a spatula to scrape down the sides as needed. Serve immediately.

**VARIATION:** You can also use cow's milk or another plant-based milk for this recipe; however, if you choose sweetened milk or use cow's milk, the carbohydrate content will increase.

**Per serving:** Calories: 284; Total fat: 16g; Carbohydrates: 32g; Fiber: 7g; Protein: 10g; Calcium: 308mg; Vitamin D: 1mcg; Vitamin $B_{12}$: 0mcg; Iron: 3mg; Zinc: 1mg

# Stovetop Granola

*Makes 4½ cups / Prep time: 10 minutes / Cook time: 10 minutes*

**ONE POT, VEGETARIAN**

Most granola is baked in an oven, but that doesn't mean it can't be made on a stove top. Using a cast-iron skillet will create a toasted flavor that mimics the baked-in-the-oven taste. The recipe itself is written as a formula, so don't feel attached to specific ingredients. Keep it simple if you feel overwhelmed by building your own recipe; just use the first recommended ingredient in the list. Serve this granola with Greek yogurt for a complete breakfast, as a topping on a salad for extra crunch, or as a smoothie garnish.

**1½ cups grains (rolled oats, rye flakes, or any flaked grain)**

**¼ cup vegetable, grapeseed, or extra-virgin olive oil**

**¼ cup honey or maple syrup**

**1 tablespoon spice (cinnamon, chai spices, turmeric, ginger, or cloves)**

**1 tablespoon citrus zest (orange, lemon, lime, or grapefruit)** (optional)

**1¼ cups roasted, chopped nuts (almonds, walnuts, or pistachios)**

**¾ cup seeds (sunflower, pumpkin, sesame, hemp, ground chia, or ground flaxseed)**

**½ cup dried fruit (golden raisins, apricots, raisins, dates, figs, or cranberries)**

**Kosher salt**

1. Heat a large dry skillet, preferably cast iron, over medium-high heat. Add the grains and cook, stirring frequently, until golden brown and toasty. Remove the grains from the skillet and transfer them to a small bowl.

2. Reduce the heat to medium, return the skillet to the heat, and add the vegetable oil, honey, and spice. Stir until thoroughly combined and bring to a simmer.

3. Once the mixture begins to bubble, reduce the heat to low and add the citrus zest (if using), toasted grains, nuts, seeds, and dried fruit. Stir and cook for another 2 minutes or until the granola is sticky and you can smell the spices. Adjust the seasonings as desired and add salt to taste.

continued

4. Allow the granola to cool before storing it in an airtight container at room temperature for up to 6 months.

**VARIATION:** Try these spice blends to encounter some new flavors. Combine in equal parts to get 1 tablespoon total for use in this recipe.

**Savory:** Red peppercorns, fennel seeds, bee pollen
**Sweet:** Cinnamon, cardamom, ginger
**Green:** Spirulina, matcha green tea powder
**Earthy:** Mushroom powder and beet powder

**Per ¼-cup serving:** Calories: 167; Total fat: 11g; Carbohydrates: 15g; Fiber: 3g; Protein: 4g; Calcium: 39mg; Vitamin D: 0mcg; Vitamin $B_{12}$: 0mcg; Iron: 1mg; Zinc: 1mg

# Seedy Muesli

*Makes 6 cups / Prep time: 5 minutes*

GLUTEN-FREE, HIGH-FIBER, NO-COOK, ONE BOWL, VEGETARIAN

A popular breakfast in Sweden and Germany, muesli consists of raw rolled grains, dried fruit, nuts, and seeds. Muesli looks a lot like granola but does not contain sweeteners or oil, so it is kinder to your heart and blood sugars. Muesli is also easier to make—no baking or cooking required. When creating your own, choose from a variety of rolled grains but avoid quick-cooking varieties because those products are less nutritious. Allow the rolled grains to soften in yogurt or milk before consuming. You'll find more seeds and nuts in this than in a classic recipe; this version has fewer carbohydrates.

**2 cups gluten-free rolled oats**
**1 cup roasted, slivered almonds**
**¾ cup raw sunflower seeds**
**½ cup raw pumpkin seeds**
**½ cup pistachios**
**½ cup apricots, sliced**
**¼ cup hemp seeds**
**¼ cup ground flaxseed**
**¼ cup toasted sesame seeds**

1. In a medium bowl, combine the oats, almonds, sunflower seeds, pumpkin seeds, pistachios, apricots, hemp seeds, flaxseed, and sesame seeds.
2. Store the mixture in an airtight container at room temperature for up to 6 months.

**SERVING SUGGESTION:** In a bowl, combine ¾ cup of muesli with ½ cup of Greek yogurt and ¼ cup of milk or milk alternative (for lower carbohydrate total) and a few fresh strawberries.

**VARIATION:** Other rolled grains such as barley, rye, spelt, or rice can be substituted for rolled oats. Try adding different spices, like a tablespoon of nutmeg, cinnamon, or both, for exciting variations!

**Per ¾-cup serving:** Calories: 430; Total fat: 29g; Carbohydrates: 30g; Fiber: 8g; Protein: 16g; Calcium: 90mg; Vitamin D: 0mcg; Vitamin $B_{12}$: 0mcg; Iron: 4mg; Zinc: 2mg

# Overnight Oats

*Serves 1 / Prep time: 5 minutes*

**GLUTEN-FREE, NO-COOK, ONE BOWL, VEGETARIAN**

Overnight oats are one of the easiest breakfasts to make: just mix and refrigerate, and then grab the finished creation as you run out the door. Not only is this breakfast effortless to make, but it also includes oats, which are a superfood because of their lower glycemic response compared with most other breakfast cereals. Oats are rich in beta-glucan, a type of fiber that reduces post-meal blood sugars and insulin responses, while delaying the absorption of carbs. This fiber also improves your gut's microbiome as a prebiotic. It's great for controlling blood sugars!

## Base Recipe

**¼ cup rolled oats, gluten-free** **¼ cup plain Greek yogurt** **¼ cup plant-based milk**

Combine the oats, Greek yogurt, and plant-based milk in a single-serving jar at least 8 ounces in size. Mix well and store overnight or for at least 6 hours. Serve with the toppings of your choice.

## Tahini, Maple, and Banana

**¼ cup plain Greek yogurt** **1 teaspoon maple syrup** **½ banana, cut into rounds**
**1 tablespoon tahini**

In a small bowl, combine the Greek yogurt, tahini, and maple syrup. Mix with the base recipe for overnight oats, put the mixture into a jar, and top it with banana. Place it in the refrigerator for at least 6 hours or overnight.

## Tropical Mango

**½ cup diced mango**

**2 tablespoons unsweetened coconut flakes**

Top the base overnight oats recipe with mango and coconut before storing it in the refrigerator for at least 6 hours or overnight.

**MAKE IT EASIER:** This dish will keep for 4 days, so double or triple the recipe and you've got yourself breakfast all week.

---

**Base recipe per serving:** Calories: 138; Total fat: 4g; Carbohydrates: 17g; Fiber: 2g; Protein: 8g; Calcium: 188mg; Vitamin D: 1mcg; Vitamin $B_{12}$: <1mcg; Iron: 1mg; Zinc: 1mg

**Tahini, Maple, and Banana per serving:** Calories: 348; Total fat: 15g; Carbohydrates: 40g; Fiber: 5g; Protein: 17g; Calcium: 330mg; Vitamin D: 1mcg; Vitamin $B_{12}$: <1mcg; Iron: 3mg; Zinc: 2mg

**Tropical Mango per serving:** Calories: 253; Total fat: 11g; Carbohydrates: 31g; Fiber: 5g; Protein: 10g; Calcium: 200mg; Vitamin D: 1mcg; Vitamin $B_{12}$: <1mcg; Iron: 2mg; Zinc: 1mg

# Apple Millet Porridge

*Serves 2 / Prep time: 3 minutes / Cook time: 12 minutes*

**GLUTEN-FREE, HIGH-FIBER, ONE POT, VEGETARIAN**

Millet is an unsung hero of the grain world—it's versatile, healthy, and delicious and yet often remains unknown. Here, millet is tastily paired with fresh apples and just a touch of honey to offer a healthy option for a warm morning meal. You will feel full and satiated all through the morning. If you have a bit more time on your hands, toast the millet by warming it up in a dry pan before starting the recipe. The natural nutty flavor will be enhanced, and it is well worth your time.

**1 cup millet, rinsed and drained**

**2½ cups plant-based milk, divided**

**2 teaspoons ground cinnamon**

**Pinch kosher salt**

**1 tablespoon honey**

**1 apple, cored and cut into bite-size pieces**

**¼ cup chopped walnuts, toasted**

1. In a small saucepan, combine the millet, 2 cups of milk, the cinnamon, and salt and place over medium heat. Cook, stirring until the millet puffs up and is fully cooked, 10 to 12 minutes.
2. Remove the millet from the heat and slowly add the remaining ½ cup of milk along with the honey. Adjust the seasonings as desired.
3. Divide the millet between two bowls and top each with half of the apple and walnuts.
4. Store any leftovers in an airtight container in the refrigerator for up to 5 days.

**SUBSTITUTION TIP:** You can substitute cow's milk in place of the plant-based milk for a creamier, richer porridge, or use water to cut back on calories and carbohydrates.

**Per serving:** Calories: 605; Total fat: 17g; Carbohydrates: 102g; Fiber: 14g; Protein: 15g; Calcium: 607mg; Vitamin D: 3mcg; Vitamin $B_{12}$: 0mcg; Iron: 5mg; Zinc: 2mg

# Breakfast Banana Barley

*Serves 2 / Prep time: 5 minutes / Cook time: 10 minutes*

**5-INGREDIENT, HIGH-FIBER, ONE POT, VEGETARIAN**

Barley is another one of the world's grains that taste great and help keep you fuller longer. Its distinct flavor enhances the sweet banana and rich peanut butter in this recipe. Barley is loaded with fiber and is typically used in soups and stews, but who said it couldn't be eaten for breakfast? It is, after all, the world's oldest cultivated cereal, grown around the globe and used as a staple in many cuisines. This dish is especially filling, so save some for a snack later if you don't finish it all in one sitting.

**3 cups water**

**Pinch kosher salt**

**1½ cups quick barley, rinsed and drained**

**3 tablespoons natural peanut butter**

**1 banana, sliced**

1. In a small saucepan, bring the water and salt to a boil over high heat.
2. Stir in the barley, cover, reduce the heat, and simmer for 10 minutes or until tender.
3. Remove the saucepan from the heat and add the peanut butter, stirring to blend. Adjust the salt as desired, and divide the mixture between two bowls.
4. Top with the sliced bananas and serve.
5. Store any leftovers in an airtight container in the refrigerator for up to 5 days.

**VARIATION:** Spice up this meal by adding some cinnamon, Chinese five-spice powder, or cardamom. This addition will really jazz up the flavor profile. Or, make it savory by omitting the banana and stirring in spinach or roasted vegetables.

**Per serving:** Calories: 725; Total fat: 14g; Carbohydrates: 136g; Fiber: 26g; Protein: 21g; Calcium: 58mg; Vitamin D: 0mcg; Vitamin $B_{12}$: 0mcg; Iron: 4mg; Zinc: 4mg

# Harvest Blackberry Quinoa Bowl

*Serves 2 / Prep time: 5 minutes / Cook time: 20 minutes*

**5-INGREDIENT, GLUTEN-FREE, HIGH-FIBER, ONE POT, VEGETARIAN**

"Bowls" are all the rage at the moment. Not only do they offer an opportunity to mix a myriad of healthy and delicious ingredients together into one satiating product, but they also allow for some creativity in the kitchen. Quinoa and blackberry, with just a touch of cinnamon, is the breakfast bowl you never knew you needed. This bowl will keep in the refrigerator for five days and can be eaten cold or hot. To reheat, simply add some liquid and zap it in the microwave for 20- to 30-second intervals until heated through, or return it to the stove top. After it's cooked, add your berries and other desired toppings.

**1½ cups water**
**Pinch kosher salt**
**¾ cup quinoa, rinsed**
**1 cup halved blackberries**
**Ground cinnamon, for garnish**

1. In a medium saucepan, bring the water and salt to a boil over high heat, reduce the heat to low, and add the quinoa.
2. Cook until you see the grains are tender and the liquid is absorbed, about 15 minutes.
3. Remove the quinoa from the heat. If you prefer your quinoa to be fluffy, then cover with a lid for a few minutes and allow it to rest. Once the quinoa is rested, use a fork to fluff it up, top it with the blackberries and a sprinkle of cinnamon, and serve.
4. If you like your grains creamier, serve immediately topped with blackberries and cinnamon.

**NUTRIENT BOOST:** If you want extra protein in the morning, consider replacing the water in the recipe with plant-based milk. Otherwise, for extra protein replace the water with cow's milk.

**Per serving:** Calories: 286; Total fat: 3g; Carbohydrates: 53g; Fiber: 10g; Protein: 10g; Calcium: 51mg; Vitamin D: 0mcg; Vitamin $B_{12}$: 0mcg; Iron: 3mg; Zinc: <1mg

# High-Protein Oatmeal

*Serves 1 / Prep time: 2 minutes / Cook time: 8 minutes*

**5-INGREDIENT, GLUTEN-FREE, HIGH-FIBER, ONE POT, VEGETARIAN**

This recipe was a part of my master's thesis in nutrition and it was the consistent favorite of all the many breakfast choices. The dish is high in protein, which is great for before or after a workout. You will find it simple and quick to prepare, and even though it is served warm, this fruit-and-nut-studded oatmeal is a great choice for any season.

**8 ounces vanilla soy milk**
**½ cup oats**
**1 tablespoon chia seeds**
**¼ cup blueberries**
**1 tablespoon sliced and toasted almonds**

1. In a medium saucepan over medium-high heat, stir together the soy milk and oats.
2. Bring to a boil, reduce the heat to low, and simmer, stirring frequently, until cooked and tender, 5 to 8 minutes.
3. Remove the oatmeal from the heat and serve topped with chia seeds, blueberries, and almonds.
4. Store any leftovers in an airtight container in the refrigerator for up to 5 days.

**VARIATION:** Instead of vanilla soy milk, use any kind of milk and a small drop of vanilla extract to get the same flavor. Another easy swap is using frozen blueberries instead of fresh. Heat the frozen berries in a separate saucepan to thaw them and serve them hot, over the oats, garnished with chia seeds and almonds.

**Per serving:** Calories: 373; Total fat: 13g; Carbohydrates: 49g; Fiber: 12g; Protein: 15g; Calcium: 420mg; Vitamin D: 3mcg; Vitamin $B_{12}$: 3mcg; Iron: 3mg; Zinc: 2mg

# Carrot Cake Oatmeal

*Serves 1 / Prep time: 3 minutes / Cook time: 10 minutes*

**GLUTEN-FREE, HIGH-FIBER, ONE POT, VEGETARIAN**

Carrot cake is one of my mother's all-time favorite desserts. However, she's allergic to eggs, so I had to come up with something special to fulfill her craving. Better yet, this dish is something she can enjoy at breakfast reminiscent of her favorite dessert. The creaminess of the almond butter with hints of sweetness from the raisins and shredded carrot will certainly remind you of the classic cake, but rest assured, this is the ideal nutritious breakfast treat.

**½ cup unsweetened almond milk**
**½ cup water**
**1 carrot, grated**
**⅓ cup rolled oats**
**1 tablespoon golden raisins**
**1 teaspoon honey**
**Pinch ground cinnamon**
**1½ tablespoons almond butter**
**½ cup cottage cheese**

1. In a small saucepan, combine the almond milk, water, grated carrot, oats, golden raisins, honey, and cinnamon over medium heat. Bring the mixture to a boil, reduce the heat to low, and simmer, stirring occasionally, until the oats are cooked, about 7 minutes.
2. Mix in the almond butter, remove the saucepan from the heat, and transfer the oats to a bowl.
3. Serve immediately, topped with cottage cheese.
4. Store any leftovers in an airtight container in the refrigerator for up to 5 days.

**SUBSTITUTION TIP:** To make this tempting breakfast vegan, substitute agave nectar for the honey and skip the cottage cheese altogether.

**Per serving:** Calories: 445; Total fat: 21g; Carbohydrates: 47g; Fiber: 7g; Protein: 21g; Calcium: 431mg; Vitamin D: 1mcg; Vitamin $B_{12}$: <1mcg; Iron: 3mg; Zinc: 2mg

# Strawberry-Ricotta Toast

*Serves 1 / Prep time: 5 minutes*

**5-INGREDIENT, HIGH-FIBER, NO-COOK, ONE BOWL, VEGETARIAN**

This dish looks decadent with sweet strawberries and rich, cloud-like ricotta cheese, but is as light and nutritious as anything else in the book. Recipes like this one illustrate just how delectable natural foods can be, and how added sugar isn't necessary for a meal that will satisfy your sweet tooth. When strawberries are out of season, choose pears or other seasonal fruit as a substitute. The ricotta cheese on the toast acts like a glue for the fruit, so make sure to dice up whichever fruit you use into small, bite-size pieces.

**2 slices whole-grain bread, toasted**

**½ cup ricotta cheese**

**2 cups diced strawberries**

**3 tablespoons toasted chopped hazelnuts**

**2 tablespoons chopped fresh mint** (optional)

1. Place the toast on your work surface and evenly divide the ricotta between the slices, spreading it out to cover the bread.
2. Top each slice with the strawberries, hazelnuts, and mint (if using), evenly distributing the ingredients on the cheese.
3. Serve immediately.

**VARIATION:** No hazelnuts on hand? Try other nuts and seeds like almonds, walnuts, poppy seeds, hemp seeds, or pumpkin seeds. Otherwise, serve it with a salad from this book.

**Per serving:** Calories: 634; Total fat: 30g; Carbohydrates: 73g; Fiber: 13g; Protein: 25g; Calcium: 465mg; Vitamin D: <1mcg; Vitamin $B_{12}$: 1mcg; Iron: 5mg; Zinc: 3mg

# Easy Buckwheat Crêpes

*Makes 12 crêpes / Prep time: 5 minutes / Cook time: 15 minutes*

**5-INGREDIENT, GLUTEN-FREE, ONE PAN, VEGETARIAN**

Traditional crêpes are very thin, cooked pancakes that originated from the northwest region of Brittany, France. As these tasty pancakes gained popularity, the recipe was revamped using wheat flour instead of buckwheat because this grain was more prevalent in many regions. When they're made into a savory version, called a galette, buckwheat flour is traditionally used. Many sweeter versions of crêpes are made with all-purpose flour, eggs, milk, and butter. What I love most about this recipe is its versatility. You can create sweet or savory crêpes with different fillings, including scrambled eggs, deli meats, cured fish, fresh fruit, cheese, nut butter, or roasted vegetables. The choice is yours!

**1 cup buckwheat flour**

**1¾ cups milk**

**⅛ teaspoon kosher salt**

**1 tablespoon extra-virgin olive oil**

**½ tablespoon ground flaxseed** (optional)

1. Combine the buckwheat flour, milk, salt, extra-virgin olive oil, and flaxseed (if using), in a bowl and whisk thoroughly, or in a blender and pulse until well combined.
2. Heat a nonstick medium skillet over medium heat. Once it's hot, add a ¼ cup of batter to the skillet, spreading it out evenly. Cook until bubbles appear and the edges crisp like a pancake, 1 to 3 minutes, then flip and cook for another 2 minutes.
3. Repeat until all the batter is used up, and the crêpes are cooked. Layer parchment paper or tea towels between the crêpes to keep them from sticking to one another while also keeping them warm until you're ready to eat.
4. Serve with the desired fillings.
5. Store any leftovers in an airtight container in the refrigerator for up to 3 days.

**MAKE IT EASIER:** If the batter starts sticking to the skillet, use a little cooking oil or spray before making each crêpe.

**Per 2-crêpe serving:** Calories: 130; Total fat: 5g; Carbohydrates: 18g; Fiber: 2g; Protein: 5g; Calcium: 89mg; Vitamin D: 1mcg; Vitamin $B_{12}$: <1mcg; Iron: 1mg; Zinc: 1mg

# Shakshuka

*Serves 4 / Prep time: 5 minutes / Cook time: 25 minutes*

HIGH-FIBER, VEGETARIAN

This is one of my absolute favorite breakfasts. It is savory and satisfying and creates an incredible choir of flavors when the garlic, harissa, and coriander harmonize with the tomato base. This recipe is influenced by the incredible food culture of Israel. It manages to be just as flavorful as anything with bacon or sausage on the side, and it's much lighter. Some versions are green, which comes from the addition of zucchini, spinach, or tomatillos (in place of the tomatoes). Throw in a handful of spinach to this recipe to boost your iron.

**2 tablespoons extra-virgin olive oil**

**1 onion, diced**

**2 tablespoons tomato paste**

**2 red bell peppers, diced**

**2 tablespoons Harissa (optional, page 169)**

**4 garlic cloves, minced**

**2 teaspoons ground cumin**

**½ teaspoon ground coriander** (optional)

**1 teaspoon smoked paprika**

**2 (14-ounce) cans diced tomatoes**

**4 large eggs**

**½ cup plain Greek yogurt**

**Bread, for dipping** (optional)

1. Heat the extra-virgin olive oil in a Dutch oven or large saucepan over medium heat. When it starts to shimmer, add the onion and cook until translucent, about 3 minutes.
2. Add the tomato paste, peppers, harissa (if using), garlic, cumin, coriander (if using), paprika, and tomatoes. Bring to a simmer and cook 10 to 15 minutes, until the peppers are cooked and the sauce is thick. Adjust the seasoning as desired.
3. Make four wells in the mixture with the back of a large spoon and gently break one egg into each well. Cover the saucepan and simmer gently until the egg whites are set but the yolks are still runny, 5 to 8 minutes.
4. Remove the saucepan from the heat and spoon the tomato mixture and one cooked egg into each of four bowls. Top with the Greek yogurt and serve with bread (if using).

**SUBSTITUTION TIP:** If you want to keep it classic and you have access to a Middle Eastern grocery store, look for labneh in place of Greek yogurt. It's creamy, slightly sour, and cheese-like. Also, consider turning up the heat and adding the optional harissa, or cayenne or red pepper flakes.

**Per serving:** Calories: 259; Total fat: 14g; Carbohydrates: 22g; Fiber: 6g; Protein: 12g; Calcium: 88mg; Vitamin D: 1mcg; Vitamin $B_{12}$: 1mcg; Iron: 2mg; Zinc: 1mg

# Eggplant Breakfast Sandwich

*Serves 2 to 4 / Prep time: 5 minutes / Cook time: 20 minutes*

**GLUTEN-FREE, HIGH-FIBER, VEGETARIAN**

Eggplant isn't a common breakfast ingredient, but this vegetable works well here as an alternative for bread. Crispy on the outside, creamy in the center, with runny egg oozing from the sides, this is a breakfast sandwich you will crave. You may want two, so plan accordingly if you are hungry or want to indulge in a breakfast that won't break the calorie bank.

**2 tablespoons extra-virgin olive oil, divided**

**1 eggplant, cut into 8 (½-inch-thick) rounds**

**¼ teaspoon kosher salt**

**¼ teaspoon freshly ground black pepper**

**4 large eggs**

**1 garlic clove, minced**

**4 cups fresh baby spinach**

**Hot sauce or Harissa (optional, page 169)**

1. Heat 1 tablespoon of extra-virgin olive oil in a large skillet over medium heat. Add the eggplant in a single layer and cook until tender and browned on both sides, 4 to 5 minutes per side. Transfer the eggplant from the skillet to a plate and season it with salt and pepper. Wipe out the skillet and set aside.

2. Meanwhile, place a large saucepan filled three-quarters full with water over medium-high heat and bring it to a simmer. Carefully break the eggs into small, individual bowls and pour slowly into a fine-mesh strainer over another bowl. Allow the excess white to drain, then lower the strainer into the water. Tilt the egg out into the water. Repeat with the remaining eggs. Swirl the water occasionally as the eggs cook and whites set, about 4 minutes. Remove the eggs with a slotted spoon, transfer them to a paper towel, and drain.

3. Heat the remaining 1 tablespoon of extra-virgin olive oil over medium heat in the large skillet and add the garlic and spinach. Cook until the spinach is wilted, about 1 minute.

4. Place one eggplant round on each of four plates and evenly divide the spinach among the rounds. Top the spinach with a poached egg on each sandwich and place the remaining eggplant round on the egg. Serve with hot sauce or harissa (if using).

**Per serving:** Calories: 362; Total fat: 25g; Carbohydrates: 21g; Fiber: 10g; Protein: 17g; Calcium: 138mg; Vitamin D: 2mcg; Vitamin $B_{12}$: 1mcg; Iron: 4mg; Zinc: 2mg

# Perfect Egg Scramble with Simple Salad

*Serves 4 / Prep time: 17 minutes / Cook time: 5 minutes*

**GLUTEN-FREE, VEGETARIAN**

This is my version of a light and fluffy egg scramble. Waiting the 15 minutes for the eggs to sit with the salt is well worth it. This method not only prevents your eggs from becoming runny on your plate, but it also enhances the taste. These eggs pair beautifully with a simple salad made with any greens you have on hand. If you don't like the spiciness of arugula, try this with leaf lettuce or mixed baby greens.

**8 large eggs**
**3 tablespoons milk**
**Kosher salt**
**6 cups arugula**
**1 tablespoon extra-virgin olive oil**
**2 tablespoons minced red onion**
**1 bunch radishes, thinly sliced**
**1 lemon, cut into wedges**
**2 tablespoons unsalted butter**

1. In a medium bowl, whisk the eggs, milk, and a pinch of salt until blended. Set aside for 15 minutes.
2. Meanwhile, in a large bowl, toss the arugula with the extra-virgin olive oil, red onion, radishes, and a pinch of salt. Evenly divide the salad among four plates and garnish each with a lemon wedge.
3. Melt the butter in a medium nonstick skillet over medium-high heat. Add the eggs to the skillet and cook by scraping the bottom very slowly, then folding. Repeat until the eggs have formed solid, moist curds. Portion the scrambled eggs evenly among the plates and serve immediately.

**MAKE IT EASIER:** Try using a mandoline to easily slice the radishes very thinly. Always use the guard that comes with this kitchen tool to protect your fingers from the blades.

**Per serving:** Calories: 262; Total fat: 20g; Carbohydrates: 6g; Fiber: 2g; Protein: 14g; Calcium: 128mg; Vitamin D: 2mcg; Vitamin $B_{12}$: 1mcg; Iron: 2mg; Zinc: 1mg

# Avocado-Tofu Scramble with Roasted Potatoes

*Serves 4 / Prep time: 5 minutes / Cook time: 25 minutes*

GLUTEN-FREE, VEGETARIAN

Crumbled tofu makes for a perfect scrambled egg replacement that's so easy to cook. The slightly curdled appearance and taste from the added spices mimic scrambled eggs quite effectively. The roasted potatoes side in this recipe is also ideal for some of the other breakfast recipes in this book. Look for colored varieties, which have more nutrients than white potatoes. Try turnips, rutabagas, or other root vegetables as healthier substitutes for potatoes as well.

**1½ pounds small potatoes, cut into bite-size pieces**

**4 tablespoons plant-based oil (safflower, olive, or grapeseed), divided**

**Kosher salt**

**Freshly ground black pepper**

**1 ounce water**

**2 teaspoons ground cumin**

**2 teaspoons turmeric**

**¼ teaspoon paprika**

**1 yellow onion, finely chopped**

**1 bell pepper, finely chopped**

**3 cups kale, torn into bite-size pieces**

**3 ounces firm tofu, drained and crumbled**

**1 avocado, diced, for garnish**

1. Preheat the oven to 425°F. Line a baking sheet with parchment paper.
2. Combine the potatoes with 2 tablespoons of oil and a pinch each of salt and pepper on the baking sheet, then toss them to coat. Roast for 20 to 25 minutes or until tender and golden brown.
3. Meanwhile, stir together the water, cumin, turmeric, and paprika until well mixed to make the sauce. Set aside.
4. Heat the remaining 2 tablespoons of oil in a large skillet over medium heat. Add the onion and bell pepper and sauté for 3 to 5 minutes. Season with a pinch of salt and pepper.
5. Add the kale to the skillet, cover, and allow the steam to cook the kale for about 2 minutes.

6. Remove the lid and, using a spatula, push the vegetables to one side of the skillet and place the tofu and sauce on the empty side. Stir until the tofu is heated through, 3 to 5 minutes. Stir the tofu and vegetables.

7. Serve the tofu scramble with the roasted potatoes on the side and garnished with avocado.

**MAKE IT EASIER:** If you have time, allowing the tofu to dry out as much as possible will make it easier to crumble it. Placing the tofu between clean kitchen towels can speed up this process considerably.

**Per serving:** Calories: 256; Total fat: 10g; Carbohydrates: 36g; Fiber: 7g; Protein: 7g; Calcium: 114mg; Vitamin D: 0mcg; Vitamin $B_{12}$: 0mcg; Iron: 4mg; Zinc: 1mg

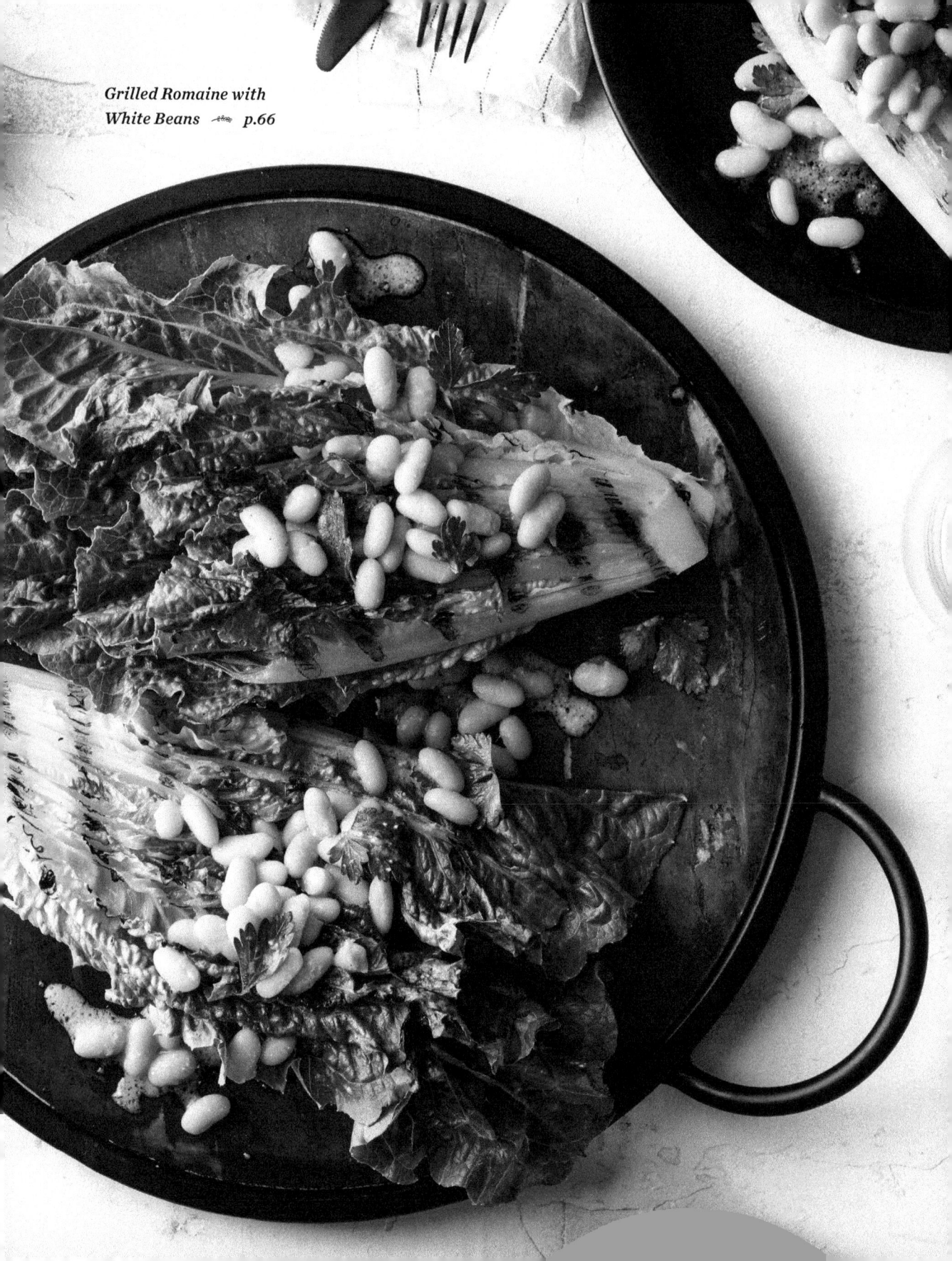

*Grilled Romaine with White Beans* p.66

CHAPTER FOUR

# Salad

Salads are often considered an afterthought, but they can be a meal in and of themselves. They're also great as a quick side, especially when trying to sneak some veggies into your meal. Salad ends up on my plate for almost every meal to help ensure I reach my recommended three to five servings per day. If the following recipes have two serving-size recommendations, the larger number applies to the dish as a side and the smaller number applies to the dish as a main. Get creative and mix and match the dressings by paging forward to the Seasonings, Sauces, and Dressings (page 157) chapter. You can also keep it simple—if you don't have a dressing handy, simply squeeze on fresh citrus juice and a drizzle of extra-virgin olive oil.

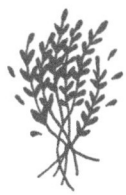

Citrus Avocado Salad ..... 55

Herbed Tomato Salad ..... 56

Spinach Salad with Strawberries and Toasted Almonds ..... 57

Asparagus Salad with Chile-Lime Dressing ..... 58

Kale Caesar Salad ..... 59

Pomegranate "Tabbouleh" with Cauliflower ..... 61

Shaved Brussels Sprouts and Kale
with Poppy Seed Dressing ..... 62

Quinoa and Cucumber Salad ..... 63

Apple-Bulgur Salad ..... 64

Sweet Beet Grain Bowl ..... 65

Grilled Romaine with White Beans ..... 66

Chickpea Fattoush Salad ..... 67

Roasted Carrot and Quinoa with Goat Cheese ..... 68

# Citrus Avocado Salad

*Serves 2 / Prep time: 10 minutes*

GLUTEN-FREE, HIGH FIBER, NO-COOK, ONE BOWL, VEGETARIAN

Looking for something bright and sunny that will leave you feeling fresh and rejuvenated? This recipe is ideal for a brunch side or for adding extra vitamin C to your day. The granola offers much-needed crunch, but it is 100 percent optional. You can substitute something else to provide the desired crispy texture like toasted pistachios, almonds, or sunflower seeds. Need more options? Serve the salad with whole-grain crackers or cooked grains.

**4 cups salad greens**

**1 grapefruit, peeled and segmented**

**1 orange, peeled and segmented**

**2 tablespoons minced red onion**

**¼ cup fresh mint leaves, torn**

**3 tablespoons Lemon Vinaigrette Dressing** (page 159) **or store-bought**

**1 avocado, thinly sliced**

**¼ cup Stovetop Granola** (optional, page 35)

In a medium bowl, toss together the salad greens, grapefruit, orange, red onion, mint, and dressing. Arrange the salad on a plate with the slices of avocado and a sprinkling of granola (if using).

**VARIATION:** Try the Tahini Dressing (page 162) or Poppy Seed Dressing (page 161) as an alternative to the lemon vinaigrette, or make prep easier by drizzling extra-virgin olive oil on top if you don't have a dressing on hand or the time to make it.

**Per serving:** Calories: 364; Total fat: 26g; Carbohydrates: 32g; Fiber: 9g; Protein: 6g; Calcium: 148mg; Vitamin D: 0mcg; Vitamin $B_{12}$: 0mcg; Iron: 5mg; Zinc: 1mg

# Herbed Tomato Salad

*Serves 2 to 4 / Prep time: 7 minutes*

**GLUTEN-FREE, NO-COOK, ONE BOWL, VEGETARIAN**

This bright and herbaceous salad is an excellent complement to the Perfect Egg Scramble (page 49) or your favorite sandwich. I look forward to tomato season all year. Tomatoes are a vibrant ingredient available year-round in the grocery store, but they are at their best late summer and early fall. They contain vitamin C, antioxidants, fiber, potassium, and folate that may help prevent cancer and support heart health.

**1 pint cherry tomatoes, halved**

**1 bunch fresh parsley, leaves only (stems discarded)**

**1 cup cilantro, leaves only (stems discarded)**

**¼ cup fresh dill**

**1 teaspoon sumac** (optional)

**2 tablespoons extra-virgin olive oil**

**Kosher salt**

**Freshly ground black pepper**

1. In a medium bowl, carefully toss together the tomatoes, parsley, cilantro, dill, sumac (if using), extra-virgin olive oil, and salt and pepper to taste.
2. Store any leftovers in an airtight container in the refrigerator for up to 3 days, but the salad is best consumed on the day it is dressed.

**SUBSTITUTION TIP:** If you don't have all the herbs listed, you can substitute other herbs, such as tarragon or mint. Most herbs taste delicious in this recipe, so use what you have on hand.

**INGREDIENT TIP:** If you have a green thumb, grow heirloom varieties of cherry tomatoes to save money. They make wonderful snacks and can quench your thirst as you wander through the garden.

**Per serving:** Calories: 161; Total fat: 14g; Carbohydrates: 8g; Fiber: 3g; Protein: 3g; Calcium: 65mg; Vitamin D: 0mcg; Vitamin $B_{12}$: 0mcg; Iron: 3mg; Zinc: 1mg

# Spinach Salad with Strawberries and Toasted Almonds

*Serves 2 to 4 / Prep time: 7 minutes*

5-INGREDIENT, GLUTEN-FREE, HIGH FIBER, NO-COOK, ONE BOWL, VEGETARIAN

Strawberry-spinach salad with balsamic or poppy seed dressing is a classic, so you have probably come across it at some point. It's a crowd-pleaser for sure, but the recipe can be improved. This is my version of the strawberry salad—with the addition of chopped toasted almonds, you get a boost of nutrition, flavor, and crunch.

**8 cups packed fresh baby spinach**

**16 strawberries, quartered**

**4 ounces goat cheese, crumbled**

**¼ cup chopped toasted almonds**

**2 tablespoons Lemon Vinaigrette Dressing** (page 159) **or store-bought**

**Kosher salt**

**Freshly ground black pepper**

1. In a bowl, gently toss together the spinach, strawberries, goat cheese, and almonds. Drizzle the salad with the vinaigrette and season with salt and pepper to taste.
2. Store any leftovers in an airtight container in the refrigerator for up to 3 days, but the salad is best consumed on the day it is dressed.

**VARIATION:** Try different greens like arugula, mizuna, mixed greens, or romaine instead of spinach or create a blend of greens for a delicious complexity in flavor and texture.

**Per serving:** Calories: 516; Total fat: 39g; Carbohydrates: 21g; Fiber: 8g; Protein: 25g; Calcium: 694mg; Vitamin D: <1mcg; Vitamin $B_{12}$: <1mcg; Iron: 6mg; Zinc: 2mg

# Asparagus Salad with Chile-Lime Dressing

*Serves 2 to 4 / Prep time: 15 minutes*

GLUTEN-FREE, HIGH-FIBER, NO-COOK, VEGETARIAN

Asparagus was proclaimed by Queen Nefertiti as the "food of the Gods," and when you taste this hearty salad, you will understand why. The elegant slender vegetable harkens the end of winter with its appearance at farmers' markets in the spring. For this recipe, you'll peel the stalks into ribbons, which you can do using a vegetable peeler. This salad highlights the addictive crunch of asparagus and the heat of the chile in the dressing. Studies suggest asparagus may also improve your body's ability to lower blood sugar naturally, so it's great to include in any meal.

**1 bunch asparagus, woody ends trimmed and stalks peeled into ribbons**

**12 ounces leftover rotisserie chicken** (optional)

**2 cups shredded cabbage**

**1 cup arugula**

**1 bunch (about 8) radishes, thinly sliced**

**½ cup mint, stemmed and finely sliced**

**3 scallions, both white and green parts, finely sliced**

**¼ to ½ cup Chile-Lime Dressing** (page 160) **or store-bought**

**⅓ cup chopped, roasted (unsalted) peanuts**

**Pickled Red Onions** (optional, page 171)

1. Combine the asparagus ribbons, chicken (if using), cabbage, arugula, radishes, mint, and scallions in a large bowl. Pour the dressing in and toss to combine with your hands or tongs.
2. Place the salad on a large serving plate and garnish it with the chopped peanuts, pickled red onions, and more chopped mint if you like.

**INGREDIENT TIP:** Prepping asparagus can take a little extra time because you have to remove the lower fibrous portion of the stalk. The best method is to bend the stalk and let it snap at the natural spot, then line up the remaining stalks and cut them at the same place.

**VARIATION:** Try using different types of cabbage in this recipe: red, green, napa, or savoy! Each variety adds a unique taste, appearance, and texture to the dish.

**Per serving:** Calories: 391; Total fat: 30g; Carbohydrates: 25g; Fiber: 10g; Protein: 13g; Calcium: 147mg; Vitamin D: 0mcg; Vitamin $B_{12}$: 0mcg; Iron: 7mg; Zinc: 2mg

# Kale Caesar Salad

*Serves 2 to 4 / Prep time: 8 minutes / Cook time: 15 minutes*

GLUTEN-FREE, HIGH-FIBER

Caesar salad is something of a staple in American restaurants. It has been prepared since Prohibition, when it was invented at Caesar's restaurant in Tijuana, Mexico. However, the traditional ingredients can be altered to create exciting new salads with the same spirit. This spin-off of the classic romaine version, featuring hearty kale instead, reminds us how versatile leafy greens can be in recipes.

### FOR THE OAT CROUTONS

**½ cup rolled oats**

**1 tablespoon sunflower seeds**

**1 tablespoon chopped almonds**

**1 tablespoon canola oil**

**1 tablespoon honey**

**Pinch kosher salt**

### FOR THE SALAD

**1 bunch kale, cleaned, ribs removed, and chopped**

**1 bunch fresh parsley, leaves only**

**¼ cup Parmesan cheese**

**¼ to ½ cup Caesar Dressing** (page 163) **or store-bought**

**1 lemon, cut into wedges** (optional)

### TO MAKE THE OAT CROUTONS

1. Preheat the oven to 350°F.
2. In a small bowl, combine the oats, sunflower seeds, almonds, oil, honey, and a pinch of salt. Toss to coat evenly, then spread the mixture on a nonstick baking sheet. Bake for 12 to 15 minutes, then remove from the oven to cool on the baking sheet for 15 minutes.

continued

### TO MAKE THE SALAD

3. Meanwhile, in a large bowl, toss the kale, parsley, and Parmesan cheese with the Caesar dressing until all the leaves are coated. Arrange the salad on plates and garnish with the lemon wedges (if using).
4. Top the salad with the croutons and serve.
5. If the dressing and oats are kept separately from the greens, then the salad and dressing will keep separately for 5 days in airtight containers in the refrigerator. The croutons will keep in an airtight container in the refrigerator for up to 1 month.

**MAKE IT EASIER:** The oat croutons are higher in protein and fiber compared to your standard crouton made from bread. If you want to forget the croutons and just eat the greens, no problem.

**Per serving:** Calories: 340; Total fat: 20g; Carbohydrates: 31g; Fiber: 6g; Protein: 12g; Calcium: 307mg; Vitamin D: <1mcg; Vitamin $B_{12}$: <1mcg; Iron: 4mg; Zinc: 2mg

# Pomegranate "Tabbouleh" with Cauliflower

*Serves 4 to 6 / Prep time: 20 minutes / Cook time: 5 minutes*

**GLUTEN-FREE, HIGH-FIBER, VEGETARIAN**

Pomegranate seeds, or arils, add a slight sweetness to this fantastic take on tabbouleh salad. Traditional tabbouleh calls for bulgur. Here, I take a bit lighter and gluten-free approach by substituting finely chopped cauliflower for the more filling grain. If you are looking for a quick late-night meal, whip this up in less than 30 minutes and enjoy. Rest assured, if you aren't worried about gluten or would prefer to use bulgur, you can substitute it for the cauliflower or add it as an extra ingredient.

**⅓ cup extra-virgin olive oil, divided**

**4 cups grated cauliflower (about 1 medium head)**

**Juice of 1 lemon**

**¼ red onion, minced**

**4 large tomatoes, diced**

**3 large bunches flat-leaf parsley, chopped**

**1 large bunch mint, chopped**

**½ cup pomegranate arils**

**Kosher salt**

**Freshly ground black pepper**

1. In a large skillet, heat 2 tablespoons of extra-virgin olive oil. When it's hot, add the cauliflower and sauté for 3 to 5 minutes or until it starts to crisp. Remove the skillet from the heat and allow the cauliflower to cool while you prep the remaining ingredients.
2. In a large bowl, combine the remaining extra-virgin olive oil with the lemon juice and red onion. Mix well, then mix in the tomatoes, parsley, mint, and pomegranate arils.
3. After the cauliflower cools, 5 to 7 minutes, add it to the bowl with the other ingredients. Season with salt and pepper to taste and serve.
4. Store any leftovers in an airtight container in the refrigerator for 3 to 5 days.

**SUBSTITUTION TIP:** Pomegranates may be challenging to find. Omit them completely or substitute diced strawberries for a similar sweet taste and pop of red color.

**Per serving:** Calories: 270; Total fat: 19g; Carbohydrates: 22g; Fiber: 8g; Protein: 7g; Calcium: 146mg; Vitamin D: 0mcg; Vitamin $B_{12}$: 0mcg; Iron: 5mg; Zinc: 1mg

# Shaved Brussels Sprouts and Kale with Poppy Seed Dressing

*Serves 4 to 6 / Prep time: 20 minutes*

**5-INGREDIENT, GLUTEN-FREE, HIGH-FIBER, NO-COOK, ONE BOWL, VEGETARIAN**

Brussels sprouts are making a comeback, but not as the notoriously overcooked army of small cabbages. They have earned their place alongside other classic greens in their raw form, as a hearty and tasty salad base. The fastest method of preparing Brussels sprouts is to use a mandoline. This kitchen utensil features two wickedly sharp parallel blades that you slide the vegetables over to produce shreds, slices, and even crinkle cuts. Be very slow and cautious with this tool, so you don't nick your finger. You can also use a knife to thinly slice the Brussels sprouts, halving them lengthwise before cutting into slices.

**1 pound Brussels sprouts, shaved**

**1 bunch kale, thinly shredded**

**4 scallions, both white and green parts, thinly sliced**

**4 ounces shredded Romano cheese**

**Poppy Seed Dressing** (page 161) **or store-bought**

**Kosher salt**

**Freshly ground black pepper**

In a large bowl, toss together the Brussels sprouts, kale, scallions, and Romano cheese. Add the dressing to the greens and toss to combine. Season with salt and pepper to taste.

**NUTRITION BOOST:** Bulk up with protein in this salad by adding hard-boiled eggs, almonds, shredded chicken, or cooked chickpeas.

**Per serving:** Calories: 251; Total fat: 12g; Carbohydrates: 23g; Fiber: 6g; Protein: 14g; Calcium: 413mg; Vitamin D: <1mcg; Vitamin $B_{12}$: <1mcg; Iron: 2mg; Zinc: 1mg

# Quinoa and Cucumber Salad

*Serves 2 to 4 / Prep time: 10 minutes / Cook time: 15 minutes*

GLUTEN-FREE, HIGH-FIBER, VEGETARIAN

Quinoa is another one of those superfoods or "super grains" that you should work to include in your diet. It's one of the few plant-based foods that contain all the essential amino acids, the building blocks of proteins that play critical roles in your body. Quinoa is loaded with protein and fiber, is gluten-free, and is a wonderful substitute for rice because it doesn't have as many carbohydrates by volume. It is also being studied for its role in diabetes and hypertension management because of its rich antioxidant level.

**1 cup quinoa, rinsed**
**2 cups water**
**Kosher salt**
**Freshly ground black pepper**
**1 bunch fresh parsley, minced**
**1 medium cucumber, cut into ¼-inch dice**
**¼ cup minced red onion**
**2 tablespoons toasted sesame seeds**
**¼ to ½ cup Tahini Dressing** (page 162) **or store-bought**
**4 ounces crumbled feta**

1. In a small saucepan, combine the quinoa with the water and a pinch each of salt and pepper. Bring to a boil over medium-high heat, then decrease to a gentle simmer and allow to cook for 10 to 15 minutes, or until the quinoa has absorbed all the water. Remove the pot from the heat, cover, and allow to rest.
2. Meanwhile, in a large bowl, mix together the parsley, cucumber, red onion, sesame seeds, and dressing.
3. Once the quinoa is fully cooked, add it to the bowl with the other ingredients. Toss to coat evenly and season with salt and pepper.
4. Top the salad with feta and serve.
5. Store any leftovers in an airtight container in the refrigerator for 3 to 5 days.

**SUBSTITUTION TIP:** Don't have quinoa? Use another grain instead. Any leftover grain will do in a pinch, such as wild rice, brown rice, quinoa, millet, bulgur, or buckwheat.

**Per serving:** Calories: 653; Total fat: 27g; Carbohydrates: 78g; Fiber: 13g; Protein: 25g; Calcium: 439mg; Vitamin D: <1mcg; Vitamin $B_{12}$: 1mcg; Iron: 8mg; Zinc: 4mg

# Apple-Bulgur Salad

*Serves 2 / Prep time: 10 minutes / Cook time: 15 minutes*

**HIGH-FIBER, VEGETARIAN**

You might have noticed an abundance of grains in this salad section. Salads are more than just greens and dressing, and adding grains turn salads into full meals that fill you up and keep you that way. This recipe uses bulgur, which soaks up the zing of vinegar incredibly well, balancing the sweet flavor of apple. Apples taste best in the autumn, when they are in season. You can plan a special outing at a local orchard to buy boatloads of apples or pick your own. If apples aren't your favorite, there are plenty of other fruits that work beautifully in this recipe, such as persimmons, kumquats, pears, grapes, or oranges.

**2 cups water**
**1 cup bulgur**
**1 teaspoon dried thyme**
**2 tablespoons extra-virgin olive oil**
**2 teaspoons cider vinegar**
**Kosher salt**
**Freshly ground black pepper**
**6 kale leaves, shredded**
**1 small apple, cored and diced**
**3 tablespoons sliced, toasted almonds**

1. In a large saucepan, bring the water to a boil over high heat and remove it from the heat. Add the bulgur and thyme, cover, and allow the grain to rest for 7 to 15 minutes or until cooked through.
2. Meanwhile, in a large bowl, whisk together the extra-virgin olive oil and cider vinegar with a pinch of salt and pepper. Add the cooked bulgur, kale, apple, and almonds to the dressing and toss to combine. Adjust the seasonings as desired.
3. Store any leftovers in an airtight container in the refrigerator for 3 to 5 days.

**VARIATION:** Add more spices for pizazz, like ground cumin or cinnamon. You can also use brown rice or quinoa in place of the bulgur.

**Per serving:** Calories: 550; Total fat: 20g; Carbohydrates: 82g; Fiber: 21g; Protein: 15g; Calcium: 157mg; Vitamin D: 0mcg; Vitamin $B_{12}$: 0mcg; Iron: 4mg; Zinc: <1mg

# Sweet Beet Grain Bowl

*Serves 2 / Prep time: 10 minutes / Cook time: 20 minutes*

HIGH-FIBER, ONE POT, VEGETARIAN

If you're not a beet person, you probably just haven't found the perfect preparation or the right variety of beet. Beets can be pickled, roasted, boiled, shaved raw into salads, pureed into soup or sauce, and even baked into bread. There are also many varieties to choose from, such as candy-cane-striped Chioggia, golden, red, and white (aka sugar beets), just to name a few. There is undoubtedly a beet for you. Here is a recipe that will surely get you hooked on these sweet, earthy, gorgeous root vegetables.

**3 cups water**

**1 cup farro, rinsed**

**2 tablespoons extra-virgin olive oil**

**1 tablespoon honey**

**3 tablespoons cider vinegar**

**Pinch freshly ground black pepper**

**4 small cooked beets, sliced**

**1 pear, cored and diced**

**6 cups mixed greens**

**⅓ cup pumpkin seeds, roasted**

**¼ cup ricotta cheese**

1. In a medium saucepan, stir together the water and farro over high heat and bring to a boil. Reduce the heat to medium and simmer until the farro is tender, 15 to 20 minutes. Drain and rinse the farro under cold running water until cool. Set aside.
2. Meanwhile, in a small bowl, whisk together the extra-virgin olive oil, honey, and vinegar. Season with black pepper.
3. Evenly divide the farro between two bowls. Top each with the beets, pear, greens, pumpkin seeds, and ricotta. Drizzle the bowls with the dressing before serving and adjust the seasonings as desired.

**VARIATION:** This recipe can be modified to include vegetables and fruits you may have on hand at home, such as carrots or parsnips. Also, you can swap out the grain for another type or add beans or lentils for more protein. This salad is an easy way to get nourished without having to think about it too hard.

**MAKE IT EASIER:** You can sometimes purchase cooked beets at the grocery store, saving you from needing to roast them at home.

**Per serving:** Calories: 779; Total fat: 29g; Carbohydrates: 108g; Fiber: 15g; Protein: 26g; Calcium: 212mg; Vitamin D: <1mcg; Vitamin $B_{12}$: <1mcg; Iron: 8mg; Zinc: 2mg

# Grilled Romaine with White Beans

*Serves 4 to 6 / Prep time: 5 minutes / Cook time: 8 minutes*

**GLUTEN-FREE, HIGH-FIBER, VEGETARIAN**

When people think of romaine, they often only picture it in salad form—chilled, dressed, maybe with a couple of croutons. Romaine on the grill is, arguably, the better way to enjoy it, and the complexity of the miso makes this plate all the more enjoyable. Miso is a Japanese seasoning paste that can be found in Asian markets but is also widely available at grocery stores. It takes years for the miso to age and finish fermenting, and this process creates a one-of-a-kind, intensely flavorful ingredient.

**3 tablespoons extra-virgin olive oil, divided**

**2 large heads romaine lettuce, halved lengthwise**

**2 tablespoons white miso**

**1 tablespoon water, plus more as needed**

**1 (15-ounce) can white beans, rinsed and drained**

**½ cup chopped fresh parsley**

1. Preheat the grill or a grill pan.
2. Drizzle 2 tablespoons of extra-virgin olive oil over the cut sides of the romaine lettuce.
3. In a medium bowl, whisk the remaining 1 tablespoon of extra-virgin olive oil with the white miso and about 1 tablespoon of water. Add more water, if necessary, to reach a thin consistency. Add the white beans and parsley to the bowl, stir, adjust the seasonings as desired, and set aside.
4. When the grill is hot, put the romaine on the grill and cook for 1 to 2 minutes on each side or until lightly charred with grill marks. Remove the lettuce from the grill and repeat with remaining lettuce halves. Set the lettuce aside on a platter or individual plates and top with the beans.
5. Serve.

**SUBSTITUTION TIP:** If you decide not to add the miso, I recommend squeezing fresh citrus or using vinegar to help replace some of the zing.

**Per serving:** Calories: 291; Total fat: 12g; Carbohydrates: 38g; Fiber: 14g; Protein: 14g; Calcium: 197mg; Vitamin D: 0mcg; Vitamin $B_{12}$: 0mcg; Iron: 8mg; Zinc: 2mg

# Chickpea Fattoush Salad

*Serves 4 / Prep time: 15 minutes / Cook time: 5 minutes*

HIGH-FIBER, VEGETARIAN

Panzanella is a Tuscan salad featuring tomatoes, onions, and heaps of stale bread cubes dressed with simple oil and vinegar. It is a lovely summer salad. Fattoush is the Levantine version of this Italian classic. Instead of bread, Fattoush uses toasted pita, chickpeas, and an assortment of mixed greens and vegetables. This recipe offers a similarly delectable salad to panzanella without nearly as many carbs.

**2 tablespoons extra-virgin olive oil**

**2 pitas, torn into bite-size pieces**

**1 (15-ounce) can chickpeas, rinsed and drained**

**1 head romaine lettuce, cut into bite-size pieces**

**1 cucumber, diced**

**½ pint cherry tomatoes, halved**

**8 radishes, thinly sliced**

**1 bunch fresh parsley, chopped**

**1 cup mint, chopped**

**½ teaspoon sumac** (optional)

**½ cup Lemon Vinaigrette Dressing** (page 159) **or store-bought**

1. Heat the extra-virgin olive oil in a large skillet over medium-high heat and sauté the pita bread until toasted and crisp, about 3 minutes. Remove the skillet from the heat and transfer the pita bread to a medium bowl.
2. Add the chickpeas, romaine, cucumber, tomatoes, radishes, parsley, mint, and sumac (if using) to the medium bowl. Add the dressing and toss to combine. Serve.
3. Store any leftovers in an airtight container in the refrigerator for up to 3 days.

**Per serving:** Calories: 466; Total fat: 30g; Carbohydrates: 42g; Fiber: 10g; Protein: 11g; Calcium: 159mg; Vitamin D: 0mcg; Vitamin $B_{12}$: 0mcg; Iron: 5mg; Zinc: 1mg

# Roasted Carrot and Quinoa with Goat Cheese

*Serves 4 / Prep time: 10 minutes / Cook time: 20 minutes*

**GLUTEN-FREE, HIGH-FIBER, VEGETARIAN**

Think of the warmth of long, lazy summer nights and the tantalizing scent of vegetables roasting. Then think of fresh, tart goat cheese with hearty, chewy grains. You just conjured up this delightful salad. Roasted carrots pair magnificently with the earthy qualities of quinoa and creamy goat cheese—this is one of those addictingly delicious salads that is full of nutrition and celebrates the natural flavors that come from the land.

**4 large carrots, cut into ⅛-inch-thick rounds**

**4 tablespoons oil (olive, safflower, or grapeseed), divided**

**2 teaspoons paprika**

**1 teaspoon turmeric**

**2 teaspoons ground cumin**

**2 cups water**

**1 cup quinoa, rinsed**

**½ cup shelled pistachios, toasted**

**4 ounces goat cheese**

**12 ounces salad greens**

1. Preheat the oven to 400°F. Line a baking sheet with parchment paper.
2. In a large bowl, toss together the carrots, 2 tablespoons of oil, the paprika, turmeric, and cumin until the carrots are well coated. Spread them evenly on the prepared baking sheet and roast until tender, 15 to 17 minutes.
3. In a medium saucepan, combine the water and quinoa over high heat. Bring to a boil, reduce the heat to low and simmer until tender, about 15 minutes.
4. Transfer the roasted carrots to a large bowl and add the cooked quinoa, remaining 2 tablespoons of oil, the pistachios, and goat cheese and toss to combine.
5. Evenly divide the greens among four plates and top with the carrot mixture. Serve.
6. Store any leftovers in an airtight container in the refrigerator for up to 2 days.

**VARIATION:** If it's summer, grill the carrots instead and consider serving the salad over plain Greek yogurt for a creamy, unique taste and texture sensation.

**Per serving:** Calories: 527; Total fat: 31g; Carbohydrates: 48g; Fiber: 10g; Protein: 17g; Calcium: 197mg; Vitamin D: <1mcg; Vitamin $B_{12}$: <1mcg; Iron: 5mg; Zinc: <1mg

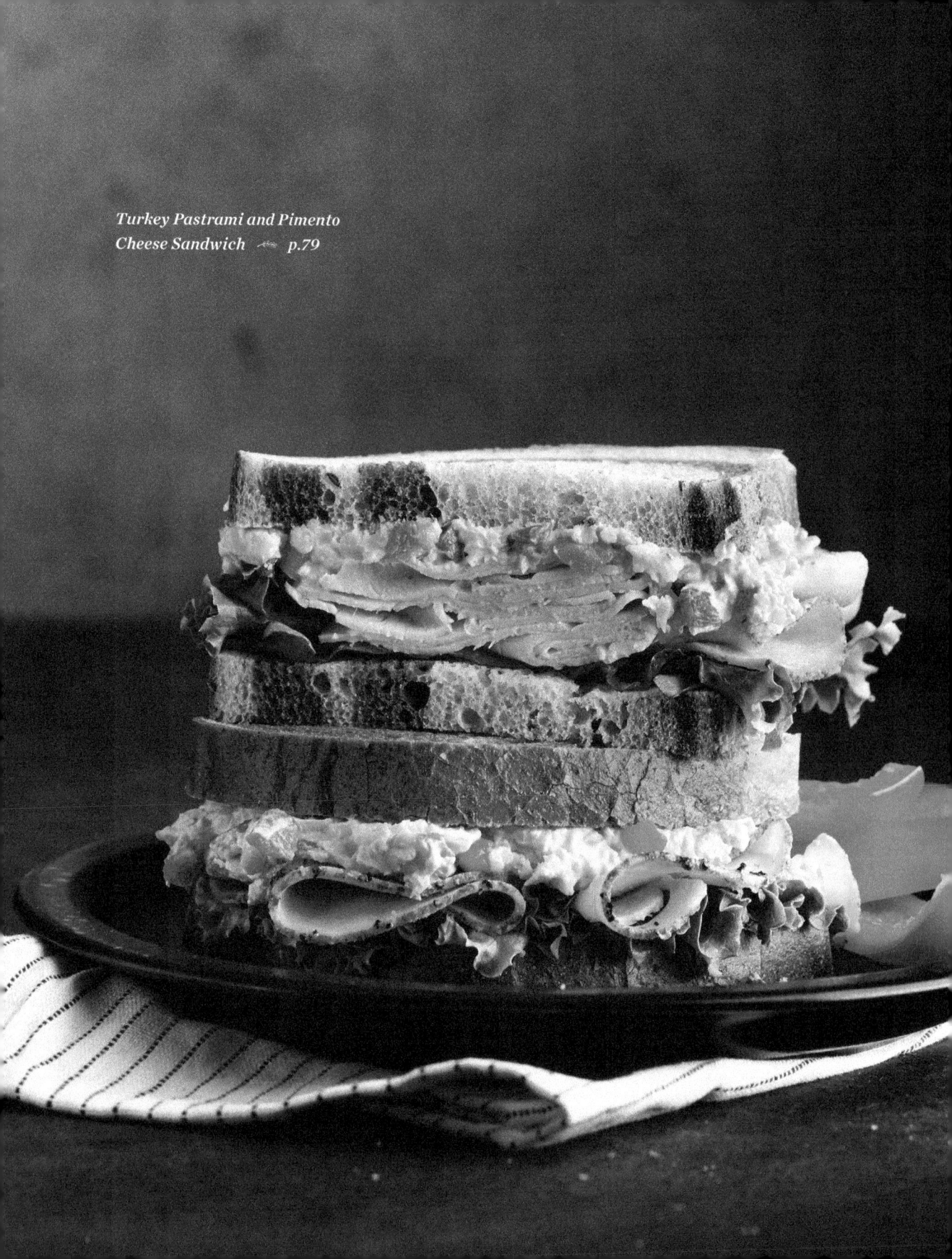

*Turkey Pastrami and Pimento Cheese Sandwich* p.79

CHAPTER FIVE

# Sandwiches and Soups

Who doesn't love a good sandwich? Sometimes it can be challenging to make sandwiches that are lower in carbohydrates. These recipes demonstrate how you can cut back on the carbs and still enjoy bread. Look for sandwich thins or flatbreads, and serve sandwiches as open-faced or tucked into lettuce leaves. Many breads are available in gluten-free varieties with the addition of vegetables such as cauliflower or spinach—or you can procure coconut wraps for your recipes.

What would a sandwich chapter be without soup, the best companion to this creation? Some soups in this section are good stand-alones; others pair beautifully with sandwiches. My suggestion is to eat less of each so that you can enjoy both.

Roasted Tomato Tartine ..... 73

Cauli-Lettuce Wraps ..... 74

Miso, Tempeh, and Carrot Wraps ..... 75

Chicken Salad with Apricots ..... 76

Smoked Salmon on Toast ..... 77

Red Lentil Sloppy Joes with Roasted Asparagus ..... 78

Turkey Pastrami and Pimento Cheese Sandwich ..... 79

Game-Day Burger with Jicama Chips ..... 80

Minted Sweet Pea Soup ..... 82

Egg Drop Soup ..... 83

Tomato-Basil Soup with Grilled Cheese Croutons ..... 84

West African–Inspired Peanut Soup ..... 86

Chickpea Spinach Soup ..... 88

Golden Chicken Soup ..... 90

Smoked Turkey Chili ..... 91

Quick Moroccan-Inspired Chicken Stew ..... 92

# Roasted Tomato Tartine

*Serves 2 / Prep time: 5 minutes / Cook time: 15 minutes*

HIGH-FIBER, VEGETARIAN

Less bread, more tomato is the equation for this delicious sandwich. This recipe goes to show that you don't have to remove bread entirely from your diet; instead, just don't eat as much. Flavorful whole-grain bread acts as a vehicle here for vibrant tomatoes, fresh basil, and tart balsamic vinegar. I like sprouted rye bread with this. If you want to add more seasonings or fresh herbs, it's up to you.

**3 tomatoes, cut into eighths**

**2 tablespoons extra-virgin olive oil, divided**

**1 tablespoon balsamic vinegar**

**2 garlic cloves, minced**

**Pinch kosher salt**

**Pinch freshly ground black pepper**

**½ cup ricotta cheese**

**2 slices whole-grain bread**

**2 tablespoons chopped fresh basil**

**4 cups arugula**

1. Preheat the oven to 450°F. Line a baking sheet with parchment paper.
2. In a medium-size bowl, toss the tomatoes with 1 tablespoon of extra-virgin olive oil, the vinegar, garlic, salt, and pepper.
3. Spread the tomatoes on the baking sheet and bake for 15 minutes.
4. Meanwhile, place the ricotta in the bowl of a food processor and, while it is running, add the remaining 1 tablespoon of extra-virgin olive oil in a thin stream. Pause to scrape down the sides if needed. Taste and adjust the seasonings as needed. If you do not have a food processor, whisk the ricotta and extra-virgin olive oil in a medium bowl.
5. Toast the bread and divide the ricotta between the slices, spreading it out evenly. Top the ricotta with the tomatoes and garnish with chopped basil.
6. Serve with the greens on the side.

**VARIATION:** Want more ricotta whip on this sandwich? Double it up on the bread or double it anyway and store the extra in the refrigerator for up to 1 week for other recipes. Adjust the seasonings with freshly ground black pepper for an even better flavor.

**Per serving:** Calories: 375; Total fat: 22g; Carbohydrates: 34g; Fiber: 6g; Protein: 13g; Calcium: 291mg; Vitamin D: <1mcg; Vitamin $B_{12}$: 1mcg; Iron: 3mg; Zinc: 2mg

# Cauli-Lettuce Wraps

*Serves 2 to 4 / Prep time: 10 minutes / Cook time: 20 minutes*

HIGH-FIBER, ONE POT, VEGETARIAN

This is a low-calorie, low-carbohydrate meal that will leave your body feeling refreshed and light. With lots of flavor and crunch, it makes for a satisfying meal that's just what the dietitian ordered to keep your blood sugars on track.

**1½ tablespoons sesame oil**

**½ yellow onion, chopped**

**8 ounces mushrooms, thinly sliced**

**4 garlic cloves, minced**

**1½ tablespoons low-sodium soy sauce or tamari**

**4 teaspoons rice wine vinegar**

**5 ounces water chestnuts, drained and liquid reserved**

**2½ cups Cauliflower Rice** (page 138)

**½ cup coarsely chopped cashews**

**4 large green leaf lettuce leaves**

**2 scallions, both white and green parts, thinly sliced** (optional)

**1 cup chopped cilantro** (optional)

1. Heat the sesame oil in a large skillet over medium heat and sauté the onion until translucent, about 3 minutes. Add the mushrooms, garlic, tamari, vinegar, and water chestnuts to the skillet. Cover the skillet with a lid and cook until the mushrooms are softened, about 5 minutes.
2. Add the cauliflower and cashews and mix well. Cover the skillet and cook for 2 minutes.
3. Adjust the seasonings as desired and evenly divide the cauliflower mixture among the lettuce leaves.
4. Serve garnished with scallions (if using) and cilantro (if using).
5. Store any leftovers in an airtight container in the refrigerator for up to 2 days.

**INGREDIENT TIP:** You can use either tamari or soy sauce here, depending on your preference; they have slightly different flavor profiles largely due to the presence of wheat.

**SUBSTITUTION TIP:** Use white vinegar or mirin if you can't find rice wine vinegar. Add a fresh chile or some chile oil if you're wanting something spicy.

**Per serving:** Calories: 413; Total fat: 25g; Carbohydrates: 38g; Fiber: 9g; Protein: 17g; Calcium: 115mg; Vitamin D: <1mcg; Vitamin $B_{12}$: <1mcg; Iron: 4mg; Zinc: 3mg

# Miso, Tempeh, and Carrot Wraps

*Serves 1 / Prep time: 10 minutes / Cook time: 10 minutes*

GLUTEN-FREE, HIGH-FIBER, VEGETARIAN

Tempeh is a fermented soy product that I use in place of animal protein. It's a wonderful, meaty protein with tons of nutritional benefits and it deserves a place in your refrigerator, especially if you're sick of using tofu. If you don't have tempeh on hand, you can substitute a couple pieces of turkey bacon or shredded cooked chicken for these light and tasty wraps.

**2 collard green leaves, washed**
**½ cup shredded carrots**
**1 teaspoon grated ginger** (optional)
**½ tablespoon white or yellow miso**
**½ tablespoon rice vinegar**
**½ tablespoon sesame oil**
**Nonstick cooking oil spray**
**4 ounces smoky tempeh, sliced**
**1 cup bean sprouts**
**4 radishes, thinly sliced**

1. Fill a large saucepan three-quarters full of water and bring it to a boil over high heat. Blanch the collard greens for 3 minutes, remove them from the water, and cool immediately under cold running water. Allow to dry and blot with a towel to remove excess water.
2. In a medium bowl, combine the carrots, ginger (if using), miso, vinegar, and sesame oil until well mixed.
3. Lightly grease a large skillet with cooking spray and heat it over medium heat. Panfry the tempeh slices until crispy on each side, about 2 minutes per side.
4. Place the collard greens on a clean work surface and evenly divide the carrot mixture, tempeh, bean sprouts, and radishes between them. Fold over the end of each leaf, tuck one side under, and roll like a burrito. Serve.
5. Store any leftovers in an airtight container in the refrigerator for up to 2 days.

**INGREDIENT SWAP:** If you want to skip the collard wraps, you could use two (6-inch) corn tortillas instead. Keep in mind that the carbohydrates will double, so consider this recipe two servings instead of one to keep the carbs low.

**Per serving:** Calories: 396; Total fat: 22g; Carbohydrates: 19g; Fiber: 6g; Protein: 31 g; Calcium: 126mg; Vitamin D: 0mcg; Vitamin $B_{12}$: <1mcg; Iron: 2mg; Zinc: 1mg

# Chicken Salad with Apricots

*Makes 4 cups / Prep time: 10 minutes*

**GLUTEN-FREE, NO-COOK, ONE BOWL**

Chicken salad, a staple of delis everywhere, doesn't have to be a bland, pale lunch staple. In fact, it becomes one of the more exciting sandwiches on our list with just a little extra spice. Dijon mustard? Sure. Coriander? Why not? And with the addition of toasted almond, parsley, lemon, and dried apricot, this filling becomes something exceptional. If you do not have cooked rotisserie chicken available, substitute canned poultry or tuna.

**1 cup plain Greek yogurt**

**2 tablespoons minced shallots**

**1 teaspoon ground coriander**

**1 teaspoon Dijon mustard** (optional)

**1 tablespoon freshly squeezed lemon juice**

**¼ teaspoon cayenne pepper**

**12 ounces cooked rotisserie chicken, shredded**

**2 cups chopped celery with the leaves**

**¼ cup slivered almonds, toasted**

**¼ cup thinly sliced dried apricots**

**1 bunch fresh parsley, chopped**

1. In a medium bowl, mix together the Greek yogurt, shallots, coriander, mustard (if using), lemon juice, and cayenne until well combined.
2. Add the chicken, celery, almonds, apricots, and parsley.
3. Serve on your food of choice (lettuce, crackers, jicama slices, radish slices—you name it).
4. Store any leftovers in an airtight container in the refrigerator for up to 3 days.

**VARIATION:** Any dried fruit can be used in place of the apricots, such as blueberries, cranberries, pineapple, mango, or golden raisins. Each will add a lovely chewy texture and balancing sweetness to the filling.

**Per 1-cup serving:** Calories: 288; Total fat: 16g; Carbohydrates: 12g; Fiber: 3g; Protein: 25g; Calcium: 135mg; Vitamin D: 0mcg; Vitamin $B_{12}$: <1mcg; Iron: 3mg; Zinc: 1mg

# Smoked Salmon on Toast

*Serves 4 / Prep time: 10 minutes*

NO-COOK

This is a classic combination for a reason, and you won't have to travel all the way to the delis of New York City to get it. Pumpernickel bread is exceptional with this recipe, but any whole-grain variety works as well. Sometimes the bread might be labeled differently, but any rye-based, thick brown bread will be fabulous. Since you're trying to cut down on your carbohydrate intake, the bread you choose to enjoy should, of course, be of the highest quality.

### FOR THE CREAM CHEESE SPREAD

**4 ounces cream cheese**

**Juice of 1 lemon**

**1 teaspoon stone-ground mustard**

### FOR THE SANDWICH

**4 slices whole-grain bread**

**8 ounces smoked salmon**

**4 radishes, thinly sliced**

**1 teaspoon capers, rinsed and dried** (optional)

**¼ cup chopped fresh dill**

**1 medium cucumber, sliced**

### TO MAKE THE CREAM CHEESE SPREAD

1. In a small bowl, combine the cream cheese, 1 teaspoon of lemon juice, and mustard. Cream together evenly and add more lemon juice if it's too thick. You should be able to spread it on a slice of bread easily.

### TO MAKE THE SANDWICH

2. Spread the cream cheese mixture on each slice of bread and top with the salmon, radish slices, capers (if using), and fresh dill.
3. Serve with cucumber slices on the side.

**VARIATION:** Substitute any cured or smoked fish such as trout, and if you really don't like fish, try cooked, thinly sliced roast beef. Beef, pumpernickel, and cream cheese are a stellar combination.

**Per serving:** Calories: 287; Total fat: 14g; Carbohydrates: 23g; Fiber: 3g; Protein: 18g; Calcium: 115mg; Vitamin D: 1mcg; Vitamin $B_{12}$: 2mcg; Iron: 2mg; Zinc: 1mg

# Red Lentil Sloppy Joes with Roasted Asparagus

*Serves 2 / Prep time: 8 minutes / Cook time: 20 minutes*

HIGH-FIBER, VEGETARIAN

This recipe is a modern take on the American classic with healthier lentils in place of ground beef. You can use sandwich thins, cauliflower thins, or serve the tasty filling open-faced; there are countless options to choose from to cut carbs. Keep it to one serving of carbohydrates, 15 grams per serving, if using the bread option, or use lettuce instead to keep those carbs in check.

**1 bunch asparagus, woody ends removed**

**1 tablespoon extra-virgin olive oil, divided**

**½ cup chopped onion**

**2 teaspoons chopped serrano pepper** (optional)

**2 garlic cloves, minced**

**1½ cups water**

**½ cup red lentils, rinsed**

**2 tablespoons ketchup**

**1 teaspoon paprika**

**1 sandwich thin or other bread option**

1. Preheat the oven to 450°F. Line a baking sheet with parchment paper.
2. In a small bowl, toss the asparagus with 1½ teaspoons of extra-virgin olive oil until well coated, and spread the vegetables on the prepared baking sheet. Bake for 12 to 15 minutes.
3. Meanwhile, heat the remaining 1½ teaspoons of extra-virgin olive oil in a medium saucepan over medium heat and sauté the onion and pepper (if using) until soft and translucent, 2 to 3 minutes. Add the garlic and cook for 1 minute.
4. Add the water and lentils and bring to a boil. Reduce the heat to low and simmer, stirring occasionally, until the lentils are tender but not falling apart, about 10 minutes.
5. Add the ketchup and paprika. Adjust seasonings as desired and allow the mixture to thicken over the heat for a couple of minutes.
6. Serve on a sandwich thin or slice of bread with a side of roasted asparagus.
7. Store any leftover filling in an airtight container in the refrigerator for up to 5 days.

**MAKE IT EASIER:** Serve with an assortment of raw veggies if you prefer to skip the asparagus.

**Per serving:** Calories: 370; Total fat: 9g; Carbohydrates: 61g; Fiber: 14g; Protein: 20g; Calcium: 129mg; Vitamin D: 0mcg; Vitamin $B_{12}$: <1mcg; Iron: 10mg; Zinc: 4mg

# Turkey Pastrami and Pimento Cheese Sandwich

*Serves 2 / Prep time: 5 minutes*

NO-COOK, ONE BOWL

The American South adopted pimento cheese, also called pimiento, depending on who you ask, over the last century, and made it their own. We use it here served with a leaner animal protein, turkey, for a sandwich that is so good it feels a bit like a cheat. The homemade pimento cheese tastes deliciously rich but is a healthier alternative to store-bought products.

### FOR THE PIMENTO CHEESE (ENOUGH FOR 4 SANDWICHES)

**6 ounces sharp cheddar cheese, shredded**

**3 tablespoons cream cheese, softened**

**1 tablespoon plain Greek yogurt**

**2 teaspoons diced pimentos**

### FOR THE TURKEY PASTRAMI SANDWICH

**4 ounces Pimento Cheese**

**4 slices marble rye bread**

**6 ounces low-sodium turkey pastrami or peppered turkey**

**4 lettuce leaves**

**1 red bell pepper, cut into strips**

### TO MAKE THE PIMENTO CHEESE

1. In a medium bowl, cream together the cheddar, cream cheese, and yogurt using a spoon.
2. Add the pimentos and stir to combine. If it's too thick, add a bit of water or pimento juice.

### TO MAKE THE TURKEY PASTRAMI SANDWICH

3. Spread the pimento cheese on each slice of marble rye bread. Layer the turkey pastrami and lettuce on the cheese spread on two of the bread slices. Place the other two slices of bread, cheese-side down, on the fillings, creating the sandwich.
4. Serve the sandwiches accompanied by sliced red bell pepper.

**Per serving:** Calories: 510; Total fat: 25g; Carbohydrates: 37g; Fiber: 4g; Protein: 31g; Calcium: 427mg; Vitamin D: <1mcg; Vitamin $B_{12}$: <1mcg; Iron: 6mg; Zinc: 2mg

# Game-Day Burger with Jicama Chips

*Serves 2 / Prep time: 5 minutes / Cook time: 22 minutes*

HIGH-FIBER

Jicama is an edible root vegetable native to Mexico, which is commonly eaten raw. It has a wonderful crunch that is reminiscent of chips—somewhere between a potato chip and a carrot stick might be the best way to describe it. And when you need something healthy and addictive alongside your burger, it is an inspired choice. After trying these lime-and-chili spiked chips, you might forget all about french fries for good.

**¼ pound ground bison**
**¼ pound ground beef**
**½ teaspoon garlic powder**
**½ teaspoon onion powder**
**½ teaspoon extra-virgin olive oil**
**1 small jicama, peeled**
**Juice of 1 lime**
**Chili powder** (optional)
**Bun** (optional)
**1 tomato, thinly sliced**
**4 lettuce leaves**

OPTIONAL TOPPINGS

**Other burger toppings (cheese, onions, mushrooms, etc.)**

1. Preheat a grill to medium-high heat.
2. In a large bowl, combine the bison, beef, garlic powder, and onion powder until mixed well. Do not overhandle, squeeze, or compress the meat.
3. Divide the meat into two equal pieces and form each into a patty.
4. Lightly oil both sides of the burger to prevent sticking and grill on the first side for 5 to 6 minutes, or until juices start to come through. Turn once and grill on the other side for another 5 to 6 minutes, or until the internal temperature is 160°F. If you want to add cheese, layer on a slice during the last minute.
5. If you do not have a grill, heat a grill pan or cast-iron skillet with 1 tablespoon of oil over medium-high heat and cook the burgers, turning once, until they reach the correct internal temperature, about 14 minutes in total.

6. Let the burgers rest 5 to 10 minutes, so the juices settle, then add the desired toppings.
7. Meanwhile, slice the jicama into 1/4-inch-thick slices, then into quarters. Put the jicama in a medium bowl and add the lime juice and chili powder (if using) to taste.
8. Serve the burgers on a bun, or wrapped in lettuce if you're watching carbs, with your favorite toppings and a side of jicama.

**SUBSTITUTION TIP:** If you can't get bison, substitute any ground meat such as pork, turkey, lamb, chicken, or more beef.

---

**Per serving:** Calories: 348; Total fat: 15g; Carbohydrates: 23g; Fiber: 11g; Protein: 32g; Calcium: 69mg; Vitamin D: 0mcg; Vitamin $B_{12}$: 3mcg; Iron: 5mg; Zinc: 7mg

# Minted Sweet Pea Soup

*Serves 2 to 4 / Prep time: 10 minutes / Cook time: 10 minutes*

**GLUTEN-FREE, HIGH-FIBER, VEGETARIAN**

I originally discovered this versatile soup recipe when looking for something refreshing to serve. I realized that peas lend themselves well to being chilled, and the addition of the mint makes for a palate-stimulating blend. This soup is just as good hot if you haven't warmed up to the idea of eating cold soup. It is an excellent side for a veggie-packed turkey sandwich or the Asparagus Salad (page 58).

**2 tablespoons extra-virgin olive oil**

**1 small yellow onion, minced**

**Pinch kosher salt**

**Pinch freshly ground black pepper**

**2 garlic cloves, minced**

**1 zucchini, diced**

**4 cups low-sodium vegetable broth**

**3 cups frozen peas**

**Juice of 1 lemon**

**½ cup plain Greek yogurt** (optional)

**½ cup thinly sliced fresh mint**

**2 tablespoons chopped pistachios** (optional)

1. Heat the extra-virgin olive oil in a medium stockpot over medium heat. Add the onion, salt, and pepper and sauté until translucent.
2. Add the garlic and zucchini and sauté until tender, about 3 minutes.
3. Transfer the vegetables to a blender and puree them with the vegetable broth, peas, and lemon juice.
4. Adjust the seasonings as desired and serve the soup warmed in a saucepan over medium heat or cooled in the refrigerator. To cool it in an ice bath, transfer the soup to a medium bowl and nestle that in a large bowl filled with ice water.
5. Serve with a dollop of optional Greek yogurt (if using) and topped with mint and pistachios (if using).
6. Store the cooled soup in an airtight container in the refrigerator for up to 5 days, with garnishes kept separately.

**SUBSTITUTION TIP:** If you don't have vegetable broth on hand, you can use water.

**Per serving:** Calories: 345; Total fat: 15g; Carbohydrates: 42g; Fiber: 13g; Protein: 12g; Calcium: 115mg; Vitamin D: 0 mcg; Vitamin $B_{12}$: 0mcg; Iron: 4mg; Zinc: 2mg

# Egg Drop Soup

*Serves 4 / Prep time: 10 minutes / Cook time: 15 minutes*

**ONE POT, VEGETARIAN**

Egg drop soup has long been a staple of Chinese buffets in the United States. This flavor-packed soup, with its whisper-thin strands of egg and light crunch of scallion, was always my childhood favorite. It is still one of my favorite cold-weather dishes, and I pay homage to those fond memories here.

**3½ cups low-sodium vegetable broth, divided**

**1 teaspoon grated fresh ginger** (optional)

**2 garlic cloves, minced**

**3 teaspoons low-sodium soy sauce or tamari**

**1 tablespoon cornstarch**

**2 large eggs, lightly beaten**

**2 scallions, both white and green parts, thinly sliced**

1. In a large saucepan, bring 3 cups plus 6 tablespoons of vegetable broth and the ginger (if using), garlic, and tamari to a boil over medium-high heat.
2. In a small bowl, make a slurry by combining the cornstarch and the remaining 2 tablespoons of broth. Stir until dissolved. Slowly add the cornstarch mixture to the rest of the heated soup, stirring until thickened, 2 to 3 minutes.
3. Reduce the heat to low and simmer. While stirring the soup, pour the eggs in slowly. Turn off the heat, add the scallions, and serve.
4. Store the cooled soup in an airtight container in the refrigerator for up to 3 days.

**INGREDIENT TIP:** Look for no-sodium or low-sodium soy sauce or tamari for this soup. Both sauces are typically high in sodium, but if you want to reduce your intake, add half the recommended amount in the recipe. Use tamari to make this recipe gluten-free.

**Per serving:** Calories: 66; Total fat: 3g; Carbohydrates: 6g; Fiber: 1g; Protein: 4g; Calcium: 40mg; Vitamin D: 1mcg; Vitamin $B_{12}$: <1mcg; Iron: 1mg; Zinc: <1mg

# Tomato-Basil Soup with Grilled Cheese Croutons

*Serves 4 to 6 / Prep time: 10 minutes / Cook time: 20 minutes*

GLUTEN-FREE (SOUP ONLY), HIGH FIBER, VEGETARIAN

Tomato soup does not have to be the pale, bland canned version; it can be vibrant and bursting with summer flavor and bright color. Fresh tomatoes are ideal for this recipe when they're in season during the summer and autumn, but there's nothing wrong with canned. Outside of this harvest time frame, fresh tomatoes tend to be mealy and mushy. If you are trying to cut down on calories, use cooking spray instead of butter to make the croutons. Make your own spray by filling a spray bottle with oil to avoid the preservatives in store-bought products.

### FOR THE TOMATO SOUP

**2 tablespoons extra-virgin olive oil**

**1 onion, chopped**

**1 tablespoon minced garlic**

**3 pounds fresh tomatoes, cored and chopped, or canned diced tomatoes**

**8 cups low-sodium vegetable broth**

**4 tablespoons tomato paste**

**½ cup coconut milk**

**½ teaspoon garlic powder**

**Pinch kosher salt**

**Pinch freshly ground black pepper**

**⅓ cup fresh basil, chopped**

### FOR THE GRILLED CHEESE CROUTONS

**1 tablespoon butter or cooking spray**

**4 slices whole-wheat bread**

**4 ounces cheese (cheddar or Gruyère), shredded**

**Freshly ground black pepper** (optional)

### TO MAKE THE TOMATO SOUP

1. Heat the extra-virgin olive oil in a medium stockpot over medium heat. Sauté the onion and minced garlic until translucent, about 3 minutes.
2. Add the tomatoes and vegetable broth, increase the heat to medium-high, cover, and simmer until the tomato skin wrinkles and pulls back from the tomato flesh, 8 to 10 minutes.
3. Add the tomato paste, coconut milk, garlic powder, salt, and pepper and simmer for 3 to 5 minutes.

4. Transfer the soup to a blender and blend until smooth, in batches if necessary. Leave the center piece out of the lid and cover the lid with a clean kitchen towel while blending to allow the steam to escape.
5. Pour the soup back into the stockpot.
6. Serve the soup topped with basil and the grilled cheese croutons (if using).
7. Store the cooled soup in an airtight container in the refrigerator for 3 to 5 days. Keep the garnishes separate.

### TO MAKE THE GRILLED CHEESE CROUTONS

8. Meanwhile, apply the butter on one side of each slice of bread.
9. Put a small nonstick skillet over medium heat, and place 1 slice of bread in the skillet, buttered-side down. Top with half of the cheese and season with pepper (if using). Then top with the second slice of bread, buttered-side up. When the underside is golden brown, 3 to 4 minutes, turn the sandwich. Cook until the second side of the bread is golden and crispy.
10. Repeat with the remaining ingredients.
11. Cut each sandwich into 1-inch squares and use them to garnish the soup.

**MAKE IT EASIER:** If you want to cut down on carbohydrates but still want the grilled cheese, use half the bread, cube it into ¼-inch-square pieces, and brown them in a skillet with 1 teaspoon of extra-virgin olive oil or fat. Sprinkle the cubes on the tomato soup followed by the shredded cheese.

**Per serving:** Calories: 230; Total fat: 13g; Carbohydrates: 27g; Fiber: 7g; Protein: 4g; Calcium: 87mg; Vitamin D: 0mcg; Vitamin $B_{12}$: 0mcg; Iron: 2mg; Zinc: 1mg

# West African–Inspired Peanut Soup

*Serves 4 to 6 / Prep time: 10 minutes / Cook time: 20 minutes*

GLUTEN-FREE, HIGH-FIBER, ONE-POT, VEGETARIAN

This soup has a complex, spicy taste and creamy, rich texture from peanut butter and coconut milk. If you are sensitive to spice, you can adjust the soup to suit your palate by removing some or all of the jalapeño seeds before mincing the pepper. Traditionally, this recipe is served over cooked rice. However, if you're trying to limit your rice consumption, use ⅓ cup of brown rice instead of a larger amount.

**6 garlic cloves, minced**

**1½-inch piece ginger, grated**

**1 jalapeño pepper, stemmed, halved, and minced, divided**

**Kosher salt**

**2 (14-ounce) cans coconut milk, divided**

**2 tablespoons vegetable oil, divided**

**1 teaspoon turmeric**

**½ cup unsweetened peanut butter**

**8 cups vegetable broth**

**2 sweet potatoes, cut into ½-inch cubes**

**1 bunch collard greens, chopped**

**Juice of 1 lime**

**Freshly ground black pepper**

**½ cup chopped cilantro**

1. Place the garlic, ginger, half the jalapeño, and a pinch of salt in a mound on a cutting board. Use the flat of your knife to create a paste. The paste can also be made in a food processor or with a mortar and pestle.

2. Scoop 3 tablespoons of the solid white coconut fat off the top of one can of coconut milk and place it in a large Dutch oven or stockpot. Add 1 tablespoon of vegetable oil to the coconut fat and heat over medium-high heat, stirring frequently, until the coconut fat separates and the solids start to sizzle, about 2 minutes. Continue cooking, stirring constantly, until the solids turn pale golden brown, about 1 minute longer. Add the garlic paste, turmeric, and peanut butter. Cook, stirring, until aromatic, about 30 seconds.

3. Add the remaining coconut milk from both cans, the broth, and sweet potatoes. Bring the soup to a boil, reduce the heat to low, and simmer until the sweet potatoes are tender, about 15 minutes.

4. When the potatoes are cooked through, use a large spoon to smash about half of the sweet potatoes against the side of the stockpot to help thicken the stew. Add the collard greens and lime juice.

5. Season the soup to taste with salt and pepper and serve topped with cilantro and the remaining minced jalapeños.
6. Store the cooled soup in an airtight container in the refrigerator for 3 to 5 days.

**NUTRIENT BOOST:** Want more vegetables in this hearty soup? Double up on the greens or add more diced yellow onion.

**Per serving:** Calories: 706; Total fat: 58g; Carbohydrates: 42g; Fiber: 8g; Protein: 13g; Calcium: 180mg; Vitamin D: 0mcg; Vitamin $B_{12}$: 0mcg; Iron: 3mg; Zinc: 2mg

# Chickpea Spinach Soup

*Serves 4 / Prep time: 5 minutes / Cook time: 25 minutes*

GLUTEN-FREE, HIGH-FIBER, VEGETARIAN

Chickpeas offer a lot of protein—you'll see them pop up more than once in this book—but they're also a fantastic ingredient because they take on the flavor of the other elements in the recipe. The texture of these legumes also combines beautifully with most accompanying ingredients. This soup makes full use of this characteristic. Take the time to enjoy how the various spices come together in this dish and discover the vibrancy of vegetarian soups.

**4 medium carrots, cut into ¼-inch pieces**

**3 tablespoons extra-virgin olive oil, divided**

**1 teaspoon ground cumin**

**1 teaspoon paprika**

**½ teaspoon ground coriander**

**½ teaspoon ground cinnamon**

**2 (15-ounce) cans chickpeas, drained and rinsed**

**1 onion, thinly sliced**

**2 tablespoons minced fresh ginger**

**5 cups low-sodium vegetable broth**

**1 pound fresh baby spinach**

**1 cup Greek yogurt** (optional)

1. Preheat the oven to 425°F. Line a baking sheet with parchment paper.
2. In a medium bowl, toss the carrots with 2 tablespoons of extra-virgin olive oil, the cumin, paprika, coriander, and cinnamon. Spread the carrots evenly on the baking sheet and roast for 8 to 10 minutes. Add half the chickpeas to the carrots, place the baking sheet back in the oven, and roast until the carrots are tender, about 10 minutes more. Set aside.
3. Meanwhile, heat the remaining 1 tablespoon of extra-virgin olive oil in a large stockpot over medium-high heat. Sauté the onion in the oil until translucent, about 3 minutes, then add the ginger, remaining chickpeas, broth, and spinach. Bring the soup to a boil, reduce the heat to low, and simmer until the greens begin to wilt, 2 to 3 minutes.
4. Transfer the soup to a blender and puree until smooth. Leave the center piece out of the lid and cover the lid with a clean dish towel to allow the steam to escape. Adjust the seasonings as desired and thin the soup with water or additional broth if you prefer a thinner soup.

5. Divide the soup among four bowls and serve topped with yogurt (if using) and the carrot and chickpea topping.
6. Store the cooled soup in an airtight container in the refrigerator for 3 to 5 days.

**MAKE IT EASIER:** If you have the spice blend ras el hanout, use 3 teaspoons of that in place of all the spices combined (cumin, paprika, coriander, and cinnamon). Sometimes it can be difficult to find, but it's a lovely spice blend.

**Per serving:** Calories: 344; Total fat: 14g; Carbohydrates: 45g; Fiber: 13g; Protein: 12g; Calcium: 157mg; Vitamin D: 0mcg; Vitamin $B_{12}$: 0mcg; Iron: 3mg; Zinc: 1mg

# Golden Chicken Soup

*Serves 4 to 6 / Prep time: 10 minutes / Cook time: 20 minutes*

GLUTEN-FREE, ONE POT

This recipe gets its name from the turmeric, an ingredient that is a staple in most people's kitchen these days. What's so special about this spice? It contains a component called curcumin that been shown to benefit inflammatory conditions, metabolic syndrome, pain, and kidney health. However, this component does not absorb well in the body unless it is paired with certain foods like black pepper. This soup contains another tasty ingredient, fennel, which has a distinct anise flavor.

**1 tablespoon extra-virgin olive oil**

**1 yellow onion, chopped**

**2 teaspoons garlic powder**

**1 tablespoon ginger powder**

**2 teaspoons turmeric**

**½ teaspoon freshly ground black pepper**

**6 cups low-sodium chicken broth**

**3 (5- to 6-ounce) boneless, skinless chicken breasts**

**4 celery stalks, cut into ¼-inch-thick slices**

**1 fennel bulb, thinly sliced**

1. Heat the extra-virgin olive oil in a large stockpot over medium heat. Sauté the onion until translucent, about 3 minutes. Add the garlic powder, ginger powder, turmeric, black pepper, and chicken broth.
2. Bring to a boil, then carefully add the chicken, celery, and fennel. Reduce the heat to medium-low, cover, and simmer until the internal temperature of the chicken is 160°F, 5 to 10 minutes.
3. Remove the chicken breasts and allow them to cool for 5 minutes while the soup keeps simmering.
4. Shred the chicken using two forks and return it to the stockpot. Heat the soup for about 1 minute and adjust the seasonings as desired.
5. Store the cooled soup in an airtight container in the refrigerator for 3 to 5 days.

**MAKE IT EASIER:** Ground ginger is less flavorful than fresh ginger, but it can be easier to use the ground product. Whichever you have, you can change out one for the other. For every 1 tablespoon of fresh ginger, use ¼ teaspoon of ground ginger.

**Per serving:** Calories: 218; Total fat: 7g; Carbohydrates: 13g; Fiber: 4g; Protein: 29g; Calcium: 56mg; Vitamin D: 0mcg; Vitamin $B_{12}$: 0mcg; Iron: 3mg; Zinc: <1mg

# Smoked Turkey Chili

*Serves 4 / Prep time: 10 minutes / Cook time: 20 minutes*

GLUTEN-FREE, HIGH-FIBER, ONE POT

Adding cocoa powder to chili was something one of the chef instructors taught me at culinary school. He also loved to add a smoky element to chili, which is why I think the adobo sauce and fire-roasted tomatoes are ideal additions as well. You can use regular canned tomatoes if you have those available instead. Make this chili ahead of time or cook it for longer to allow for a richer, deeper flavor. All good meaty stews develop complex flavor over time.

**1 tablespoon extra-virgin olive oil**

**1 yellow onion, diced**

**2 bell peppers, diced**

**½ pound ground turkey**

**1½ teaspoons ground cumin**

**1 teaspoon ground coriander**

**1 tablespoon cocoa powder** (optional)

**3 tablespoons adobo sauce**

**1 cup low-sodium chicken or vegetable broth**

**1 (28-ounce) can crushed fire-roasted tomatoes**

**2 (15-ounce) cans cooked beans (kidney beans, black beans, or navy beans), rinsed and drained**

1. Heat the extra-virgin olive oil in a large stockpot over medium-high heat. Add the onion and bell peppers and sauté until softened, about 5 minutes.
2. Add the ground turkey and sauté until cooked through, 3 to 5 minutes. Add the cumin, coriander, cocoa powder (if using), and adobo sauce. Stir well and add the broth, tomatoes, and beans.
3. Bring to a boil, reduce the heat to low, and simmer for at least 15 minutes. The longer you have, the better the flavors will be enhanced. Serve.
4. Store the cooled chili in an airtight container in the refrigerator for 3 to 5 days.

**VARIATION:** Replace the ground turkey with 1 cup of quinoa or 2 cups cubed of butternut squash and use the vegetable broth if you'd prefer to make this chili vegan. These substitutions will take about 15 minutes to cook and can be added after you've sautéed the onions and vegetables.

**Per serving:** Calories: 329; Total fat: 12g; Carbohydrates: 37g; Fiber: 13g; Protein: 19g; Calcium: 93mg; Vitamin D: <1mcg; Vitamin $B_{12}$: 1mcg; Iron: 4mg; Zinc: 2mg

# Quick Moroccan-Inspired Chicken Stew

*Serves 4 to 6 / Prep time: 5 minutes / Cook time: 15 minutes*

**GLUTEN-FREE, ONE POT**

The inspiration behind this recipe comes from a Moroccan cooking class I teach regularly. Traditionally, this recipe is made using a tagine, an earthenware cooking vessel popular in North Africa. You can substitute a Dutch oven or use a large pan with a lid to capture the moisture. This is a sped-up version of the classic recipe. If you have the time, extend the cooking time once all the ingredients are combined to create a rich, deeply flavored stew.

**2 teaspoons ground cumin**

**1 teaspoon ground cinnamon**

**½ teaspoon turmeric**

**½ teaspoon paprika**

**1½ pounds boneless, skinless chicken, cut into strips**

**2 tablespoons extra-virgin olive oil**

**5 garlic cloves, smashed and coarsely chopped**

**2 onions, thinly sliced**

**1 tablespoon fresh lemon zest**

**½ cup coarsely chopped olives**

**2 cups low-sodium chicken broth**

**Cilantro, for garnish** (optional)

1. In a medium bowl, mix together the cumin, cinnamon, turmeric, and paprika until well blended. Add the chicken, tossing to coat, and set aside.
2. Heat the extra-virgin olive oil in a large skillet or medium Dutch oven over medium-high heat. Add the chicken and garlic in one layer and cook, browning on all sides, about 2 minutes.
3. Add the onions, lemon zest, olives, and broth and bring the soup to a boil. Reduce the heat to medium low, cover, and simmer for 8 minutes.
4. Uncover the soup and let it simmer for another 2 to 3 minutes for the sauce to thicken slightly. Adjust the seasonings as desired and serve garnished with cilantro (if using).
5. Store the cooled soup in an airtight container in the refrigerator for up to 5 days.

**VARIATION:** Make this stew vegetarian by omitting the chicken and adding cooked chickpeas. Also, swap out the chicken broth for a vegetarian product.

**Per serving:** Calories: 315; Total fat: 14g; Carbohydrates: 9g; Fiber: 2g; Protein: 40g; Calcium: 55mg; Vitamin D: 0mcg; Vitamin $B_{12}$: 0mcg; Iron: 3mg; Zinc: <1mg

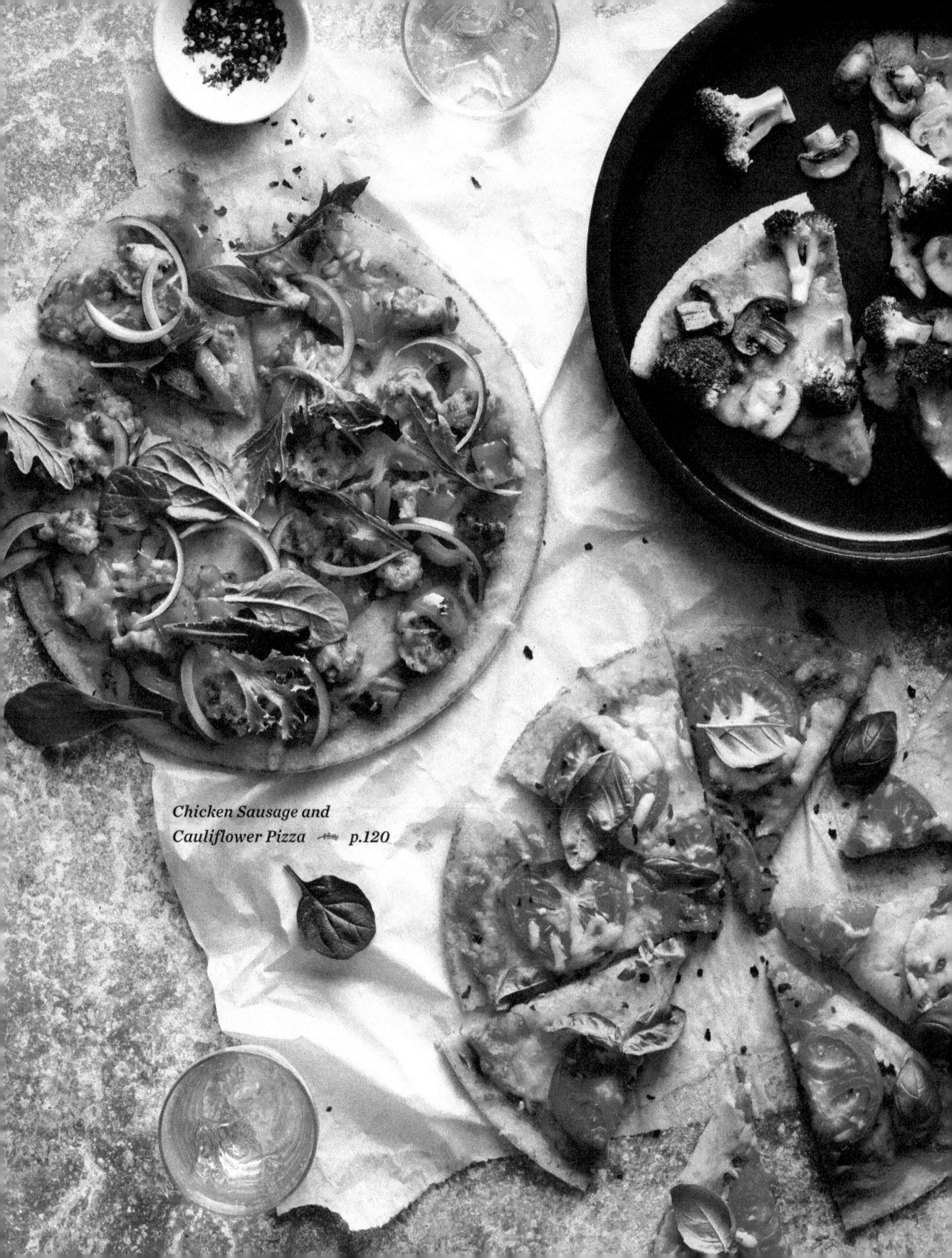

*Chicken Sausage and Cauliflower Pizza* p.120

CHAPTER SIX

# Mains

Our culture reveres big plates and 16-ounce steaks. We've long held the view that large portions are the only prerequisite for being called the main course. While I want to ensure that you remain satiated—no one who follows the recipes in this cookbook will go to bed hungry—this mentality couldn't be further from the truth. Having the *right* items on your plate, as opposed to a mountain of empty calories or extra-large portions, is infinitely more important.

The main courses in this chapter draw inspiration from all over the world and lean into lighter, healthier vegetable replacements for meats. You might be surprised at how many of your favorites can be found in this book. I also draw from the cuisines of other countries and cultures to ensure a balanced diet that incorporates everything you need to expand your horizons while eating healthy to boot.

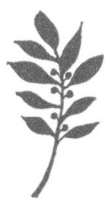

Gingered Red Lentils with Millet ..... 97

Eggplant and Lentils with Curried Yogurt ..... 98

Peanut Tofu over Buckwheat Noodles ..... 100

Simple Bibimbap ..... 101

Vegetable Mac 'n' Cheese ..... 102

Jackfruit Tacos ..... 103

Cauliflower Steaks with Tomato, Caper, and Golden Raisin Sauce ..... 104

Tuna Poke with Riced Broccoli ..... 105

Walnut-Crusted Halibut with Pear Salad ..... 107

Italian-Style Turkey Meatballs and Zoodles ..... 109

Ribboned Squash with Bacon ..... 110

Chicken Khao Sen with Rice Noodles ..... 111

Lebanese-Inspired Beef Kebabs with Pickled Onions ..... 112

Salmon en Papillote ..... 114

Cherry Barbecue Chicken Cutlets ..... 116

Miso Skirt Steak ..... 118

Herbed Buttermilk Chicken ..... 119

Chicken Sausage and Cauliflower Pizza ..... 120

Turkey Bolognese with Chickpea Pasta ..... 121

# Gingered Red Lentils with Millet

*Serves 4 / Prep time: 10 minutes / Cook time: 20 minutes*

**GLUTEN-FREE, HIGH-FIBER, VEGETARIAN**

This recipe is inspired by the delicious cuisine of India—where it would be called *dal*. One of my favorite food countries, India, has long ago mastered the art of balanced eating, with the understanding that you don't have to sacrifice great, bold flavors to enjoy vegetarian food. You will find the blend of ginger, mint, onions, and tomato in this dish is, in a word, perfect.

**3 cups water**

**1 cup millet, rinsed**

**½ cup red lentils, rinsed**

**3 tablespoons extra-virgin olive oil, divided**

**Pinch kosher salt**

**1 onion, diced**

**3-inch piece ginger, grated (or minced)**

**4 cups cherry tomatoes, diced**

**3 tablespoons unsalted peanuts, chopped**

**2 limes, quartered**

**1 bunch mint leaves**

1. In a medium saucepan over medium heat, stir together the water, millet, lentils, 1 tablespoon of extra-virgin olive oil, and the salt. Bring to a boil, reduce the heat to low, cover, and simmer until tender, about 15 minutes. Remove the saucepan from the heat and let the grains sit for a few minutes.

2. Meanwhile, in a small saucepan, heat the remaining 2 tablespoons of extra-virgin olive oil. Sauté the onion until translucent, about 3 minutes. Add the ginger, tomatoes, and peanuts. Cook for about 5 minutes, adjust the seasonings as desired, and allow to sit until the millet and lentils are finished.

3. Divide the millet and lentils among four bowls, and top them with the gingered onion mixture. Garnish with lime wedges and mint leaves.

4. Serve, and store any leftovers in an airtight container in the refrigerator for up to 3 days.

**MAKE IT EASIER:** Only want to cook for two? Simply use half the ingredients or pack up the leftovers in an airtight container in the refrigerator to enjoy another day.

**Per serving:** Calories: 439; Total fat: 16g; Carbohydrates: 62g; Fiber: 8g; Protein: 15g; Calcium: 46mg; Vitamin D: 0mcg; Vitamin $B_{12}$: 0mcg; Iron: 5mg; Zinc: 1mg

# Eggplant and Lentils with Curried Yogurt

*Serves 4 / Prep time: 10 minutes / Cook time: 20 minutes*

GLUTEN-FREE, HIGH-FIBER, VEGETARIAN

My partner has perfected this flavorful recipe. He can get anyone to eat eggplant when he prepares this dish, and it is definitely a crowd-pleasing recipe that's enjoyed above any other at our friend's potluck dinners. If you have the time before you begin cooking, soaking the lentils for 1 hour before preparing this dish helps shorten the cooking time.

**2 large eggplants**

**4 tablespoons extra-virgin olive oil, divided**

**Kosher salt**

**2 cups water**

**1 cup brown lentils, rinsed and soaked (optional to soak)**

**1 teaspoon ground cumin, divided**

**¾ cup plain Greek yogurt**

**2 teaspoons curry powder**

**Zest and juice of 1 lime**

**1 onion, thinly sliced**

**¼ cup sliced almonds**

**½ teaspoon ground coriander**

**¼ cup pomegranate seeds**

1. Preheat the oven to 450°F. Line a baking sheet with parchment paper.
2. Use a peeler to peel strips of the skin off of the eggplant lengthwise. Alternate strips, leaving some of the purplish-black skin on the eggplant. It should be reminiscent of a zebra with the white flesh and dark skin. Cut the peeled eggplant width-wise into ½-inch-thick slices. Place them in a medium bowl.
3. Toss the eggplant with 2 tablespoons of extra-virgin olive oil and a pinch of salt. Spread the slices in a single layer on the prepared baking sheet. Roast the eggplant for 20 minutes, until slightly crispy and soft.
4. Meanwhile, in a medium stockpot over medium-high heat, combine the water, lentils, ½ teaspoon of cumin, and a pinch of salt. Bring to a boil, then reduce the heat to low, cover, and simmer for 20 minutes or until the lentils are tender. Set aside.

5. In a small bowl, combine the Greek yogurt with the curry powder, a pinch of lime zest, and 1 tablespoon of lime juice. Taste and adjust the seasonings as desired. Use the additional lime juice if you feel it should have more citrus or a looser consistency. Set aside.

6. Heat the remaining 2 tablespoons of extra-virgin olive oil in a medium skillet over medium-high heat. Sauté the onion until translucent, about 3 minutes. Add the remaining ½ teaspoon of cumin, the sliced almonds, and coriander to the skillet, stirring to combine.

7. Arrange the slices of eggplant on four plates, followed by the lentils, spiced yogurt, sautéed onions, and garnish with pomegranate seeds.

**SUBSTITUTION TIP:** You can use dried cherries or dried cranberries in place of the pomegranate seeds, if preferred.

**Per serving:** Calories: 479; Total fat: 20g; Carbohydrates: 56g; Fiber: 27g; Protein: 23g; Calcium: 161mg; Vitamin D: 0mcg; Vitamin $B_{12}$: <1mcg; Iron: 5mg; Zinc: 1mg

# Peanut Tofu over Buckwheat Noodles

*Serves 2 / Prep time: 5 to 10 minutes / Cook time: 10 minutes*

**GLUTEN-FREE, HIGH-FIBER, ONE POT, VEGETARIAN**

This delightful recipe is loaded with veggies, enough for your entire day, as well as deliciously thick buckwheat noodles. Yes, you can eat noodles if you're a diabetic or are trying to limit your carbohydrates; this recipe simply ensures that you're not getting too much of a good thing.

**2 ounces buckwheat noodles**

**¼ cup Peanut Sauce** (page 168) **or store-bought**

**4 cups shredded cabbage**

**8 ounces firm tofu, cubed**

**1 cup diced cucumber**

**½ cup chopped cilantro**

1. Cook the buckwheat noodles according to the package instructions and allow to cool. This can be done 1 to 2 days in advance, and you can store the cooked noodles in the refrigerator in an airtight container.
2. In a large bowl, thin the peanut sauce with water if it's too thick. It should resemble the consistency of a thin dressing. Toss the sauce with the noodles, cabbage, tofu, cucumber, and cilantro. Adjust the seasonings as desired. Serve.
3. Store any leftovers in an airtight container in the refrigerator for up to 3 days.

**MAKE IT EASIER:** If you like extra sauce, double up on the peanut sauce. It will increase your protein and fat to keep you fuller longer.

**SUBSTITUTION TIP:** If you're not a fan of cilantro, you can use equal amounts of parsley, any lettuce, red cabbage, or shredded carrot instead.

**Per serving:** Calories: 462; Total fat: 23g; Carbohydrates: 45g; Fiber: 8g; Protein: 26g; Calcium: 277mg; Vitamin D: 0mcg; Vitamin $B_{12}$: 0mcg; Iron: 4mg; Zinc: 1mg

# Simple Bibimbap

*Serves 2 / Prep time: 15 minutes / Cook time: 15 minutes*

**HIGH-FIBER, VEGETARIAN**

Korean bibimbap ("bibim" means to mix various ingredients and "bap" means rice) is the ultimate casual meal. I've formulated one of my favorite combinations here, but feel free to experiment with the extra veggies and sauces you have in the refrigerator as well. The cauliflower rice helps you cut back on the concentrated carbs of traditional rice, and kimchi is a delicious good-for-your-gut probiotic food that helps with digestion and immunity. You can find it at many grocery stores in the international aisle.

**4 teaspoons canola oil, divided**

**2½ cups Cauliflower Rice** (page 138)

**2 cups fresh baby spinach**

**3 teaspoons low-sodium soy sauce or tamari, divided**

**8 ounces mushrooms, thinly sliced**

**2 large eggs**

**1 cup bean sprouts, rinsed**

**1 cup kimchi**

**½ cup shredded carrots**

1. Heat 1 teaspoon of canola oil in a medium skillet and sauté the cauliflower rice, spinach, and 2 teaspoons of soy sauce until the greens are wilted, about 5 minutes. Put the vegetables in a small bowl and set aside.
2. Return the skillet to medium heat, add 2 teaspoons of vegetable oil and, when it's hot, add the mushrooms in a single layer and cook for 3 to 5 minutes, then stir and cook another 3 minutes or until mostly golden-brown in color. Put the mushrooms in a small bowl and toss them with the remaining 1 teaspoon of soy sauce.
3. Wipe out the skillet and heat the remaining 1 teaspoon of vegetable oil over low heat. Crack in the eggs and cook until the whites are set and the yolks begin to thicken but not harden, 4 to 5 minutes.
4. Assemble two bowls with cauliflower rice and spinach at the bottom. Then arrange each ingredient separately around the rim of the bowl: bean sprouts, mushrooms, kimchi, and shredded carrots, with the egg placed in the center, and serve.

**NUTRIENT BOOST:** Add some sliced radishes for more vegetables, or serve with whole grains.

**Per serving:** Calories: 277; Total fat: 15g; Carbohydrates: 20g; Fiber: 8g; Protein: 18g; Calcium: 164mg; Vitamin D: 1mcg; Vitamin $B_{12}$: 1mcg; Iron: 3mg; Zinc: 2mg

# Vegetable Mac 'n' Cheese

*Serves 2 / Prep time: 10 minutes / Cook time: 20 minutes*

HIGH-FIBER, VEGETARIAN

The "comfort food revolution," which introduced items like burgers and tater tots to fine-dining menus all across the country, thankfully also convinced us that macaroni and cheese is not just for children. We limit the pasta shells here and bolster the dish with cauliflower and Brussels sprouts to make this lower-carb and suitable for prediabetes.

**2 cups Brussels sprouts, quartered**

**1 tablespoon extra-virgin olive oil, divided**

**Pinch kosher salt**

**Pinch freshly ground black pepper**

**¼ cup dry whole-wheat pasta shells**

**½ cup sliced leeks**

**2 cups small cauliflower florets**

**4 ounces shredded cheddar cheese**

**2 tablespoons milk**

1. Preheat the oven to 425°F. Line a baking sheet with parchment paper.
2. In a large bowl, toss the Brussels sprouts in 2 teaspoons of extra-virgin olive oil, the salt, and pepper. Arrange the sprouts on the prepared baking sheet and roast for 20 minutes, until softened and browned.
3. Meanwhile, bring a medium saucepan filled three-quarters full of water to a boil over high heat and cook the pasta according to the package instructions. Drain and set aside.
4. Heat the remaining 1 teaspoon of extra-virgin olive oil in a medium saucepan over medium-high heat and sauté the leeks until translucent, about 3 minutes. Add the cauliflower, cheese, milk, and cooked pasta. Stir until the mixture has a creamy consistency. Add the Brussels sprouts and toss to combine before serving.
5. Store any leftovers in an airtight container in the refrigerator for up to 4 days.

**SUBSTITUTION TIP:** Don't let the leeks stop you from making this recipe if you can't find them. Use any onion you'd like as a substitute. You can toss in some kimchi for a Korean take on mac 'n' cheese as well. It's delicious, trust me.

**Per serving:** Calories: 401; Total fat: 26g; Carbohydrates: 26g; Fiber: 8g; Protein: 21g; Calcium: 481mg; Vitamin D: <1mcg; Vitamin $B_{12}$: <1mcg; Iron: 2mg; Zinc: 1mg

# Jackfruit Tacos

*Serves 4 / Prep time: 5 minutes / Cook time: 25 minutes*

GLUTEN-FREE, HIGH-FIBER, VEGETARIAN

You may have heard of jackfruit as the go-to meat substitute. Not only does it have a succulent, pulled pork–like texture, but it also takes on the flavor and spice of ingredients it's cooked with. Surprisingly, jackfruit is actually best canned as opposed to raw. You can find it in Asian markets or the international aisle of your grocery store.

**2 (20-ounce) cans jackfruit in water, rinsed and drained**

**2 tablespoons extra-virgin olive oil**

**1 yellow onion, diced**

**1 cup water**

**4 garlic cloves, minced**

**2 teaspoons paprika**

**1 tablespoon chili powder**

**1 tablespoon ground cumin**

**1 chipotle pepper in adobo sauce, minced, plus 2 tablespoons sauce**

**Juice of 2 limes**

OPTIONAL TOPPINGS

**Corn tortillas**

**Shredded cabbage or lettuce**

**Cheese**

**Salsa**

**Cooked beans**

**Avocado**

1. Place the jackfruit in a medium bowl. Sort through it and cut the tougher core portion of the jackfruit into smaller pieces. Use your hands to break up some of the larger, tender pieces. Pat dry and set aside.
2. Heat the extra-virgin olive oil in a large skillet over medium heat and sauté the onion until translucent, 3 to 5 minutes. Add the jackfruit, water, garlic, paprika, chili powder, cumin, chipotle pepper and adobo sauce, and lime juice. Mix well, reduce the heat to medium-low, cover, and cook, stirring occasionally, for 15 minutes.
3. Serve with corn tortillas, lettuce or cabbage, and any other taco additions you see fit.
4. Store any leftovers in an airtight container in the refrigerator for up to 4 days.

**VARIATION:** Make this recipe a salad by placing the filling components on a bed of fresh greens or Avocado Slaw (page 142).

**Per serving:** Calories: 139; Total fat: 8g; Carbohydrates: 18g; Fiber: 10g; Protein: 2g; Calcium: 71mg; Vitamin D: 0mcg; Vitamin $B_{12}$: 0mcg; Iron: 1mg; Zinc: <1mg

# Cauliflower Steaks with Tomato, Caper, and Golden Raisin Sauce

*Serves 4 / Prep time: 5 minutes / Cook time: 25 minutes*

**5-INGREDIENT, GLUTEN-FREE, HIGH FIBER, VEGETARIAN**

I was once skeptical about cauliflower steaks as a swap for animal protein, but they're quite delicious! It is the stellar sauce that really makes this dish shine. The combination of tomatoes, capers, and golden raisins with cauliflower creates an Italian-influenced plate that lingers in your memory long after the last bite.

**1 large head cauliflower**

**2 tablespoons extra-virgin olive oil**

**Pinch kosher salt**

**Pinch freshly ground black pepper**

**1 batch Tomato, Caper, and Golden Raisin Sauce** (page 167)

1. Preheat the oven to 400°F. Line a baking sheet with parchment paper.
2. Stand up the cauliflower so that the stem end is flat on the cutting board while you hold the crown of the head with your hand. Then, carefully, slice ½-inch-thick "steaks" starting from the crown (top of the head) and moving toward the stem (base). Work from one end to the other. Depending on the size of the cauliflower, you should get 4 to 6 sliced steaks and some florets.
3. Place the cauliflower steaks and florets on the prepared baking sheet in a single layer. Brush them with oil and season with salt and pepper.
4. Roast the cauliflower for 15 minutes until golden brown, then flip the steaks over and cook for another 10 minutes.
5. To serve, lay the cauliflower steaks on plates and top with the tomato sauce.
6. Store any leftovers in an airtight container in the refrigerator for up to 4 days.

**MAKE IT EASIER:** If you really want to cut down on the cooking time, you can always use a canned tomato sauce instead of making the tomato-caper sauce. Simply heat the sauce in a saucepan on the stove until warm.

**Per serving:** Calories: 275; Total fat: 15g; Carbohydrates: 35g; Fiber: 9g; Protein: 8g; Calcium: 139mg; Vitamin D: 0mcg; Vitamin $B_{12}$: 0mcg; Iron: 4mg; Zinc: 1mg

# Tuna Poke with Riced Broccoli

*Serves 2 / Prep time: 15 minutes / Cook time: 5 minutes*

HIGH-FIBER, ONE PAN

Instead of having rice in your tuna poke bowl, try riced broccoli, your favorite green mini trees. You may be able to find riced broccoli at the store, but it's actually quite easy to prep at home. Simply grate raw broccoli, and that's it! It's loaded with fiber; vitamins C, E, and K; and minerals like folate, calcium, and potassium. It also won't affect your blood sugars like starchy grains. Another option is to use Cauliflower Rice (page 138) if broccoli isn't an ingredient you're keen on.

### FOR THE TUNA POKE

**½ pound sushi-grade tuna (see tip), cut into ½-inch cubes**

**2 tablespoons soy sauce or tamari**

**1 tablespoon rice vinegar**

**1 teaspoon sesame oil**

### FOR THE BOWL

**½ tablespoon extra-virgin olive oil**

**1 small head broccoli, grated**

**1 cup thawed (if frozen) edamame**

**1 medium carrot, julienned**

**1 cucumber, diced**

**2 scallions, both white and green parts, thinly sliced**

### OPTIONAL TOPPINGS

**Avocado slices**

**Shaved radish**

**Toasted sesame seeds**

**Pickled ginger**

### TO MAKE THE TUNA POKE

1. In a medium bowl, toss together the tuna, soy sauce, rice vinegar, and sesame oil.
2. Set aside.

continued

### TO MAKE THE BOWL

3. Heat the oil in a large skillet over medium heat and sauté the broccoli until tender, 2 to 3 minutes. Remove the skillet from the heat and allow the broccoli to cool.
4. Assemble two bowls by placing riced broccoli as the base. Top each bowl with the tuna poke, edamame, carrot, and cucumber. Drizzle the remaining juices from the tuna marinade over the bowls and garnish with sliced scallions.
5. Store any leftovers in an airtight container in the refrigerator for up to 2 days.

**SUBSTITUTION TIP:** Make it a budget tuna poke bowl by using canned tuna instead of fresh. Drain the tuna before adding the seasonings and follow the recipe as instructed.

**Per serving:** Calories: 374; Total fat: 11g; Carbohydrates: 28g; Fiber: 10g; Protein: 46g; Calcium: 179mg; Vitamin D: 3mcg; Vitamin $B_{12}$: 0mcg; Iron: 4mg; Zinc: 1mg

# Walnut-Crusted Halibut with Pear Salad

*Serves 4 / Prep time: 10 minutes / Cook time: 10 minutes*

HIGH-FIBER

Halibut is one of my favorite types of whitefish, but another whitefish, such as cod, can be a tasty substitute. Whatever the fish you decide to use, your heart still benefits from the lean protein and healthy fats it has to offer. Additionally, fish is low in carbohydrates and high in protein, especially paired with those non-starchy vegetables you just can't get enough of.

### FOR THE HALIBUT

**¾ cup finely chopped toasted walnuts**

**2 tablespoons bread crumbs**

**¼ cup chopped fresh parsley**

**2 tablespoons chopped fresh chives**

**4 (6- to 8-ounce) halibut fillets**

**Kosher salt**

**Freshly ground black pepper**

**1 tablespoon extra-virgin olive oil**

### FOR THE SALAD

**6 cups packed mixed greens**

**1 pear, thinly sliced**

**¼ cup chopped fresh parsley**

**¼ cup chopped fresh chives**

**Zest and juice of 1 lemon**

**Extra-virgin olive oil, for the dressing**

**Kosher salt**

**Freshly ground black pepper**

### TO MAKE THE HALIBUT

1. Preheat the broiler. Line a baking sheet with parchment paper.
2. In a small bowl, combine the walnuts, bread crumbs, parsley, and chives.
3. Pat the halibut fillets dry, season them with salt and pepper and rub ½ tablespoon of extra-virgin olive oil on each fillet. Place the fillets on the prepared baking sheet. Sprinkle the walnut mixture evenly on top of each fillet and press slightly, so the topping will stick.
4. Broil the fish until the crust is golden and the fish is fully cooked, 5 to 8 minutes.

continued

### TO MAKE THE SALAD

5. Meanwhile, in a large bowl, toss the greens, pear, parsley, chives, and zest until well combined. Drizzle the salad with the lemon juice and a bit of extra-virgin olive oil to taste. Season with salt and pepper to taste.
6. Evenly divide the salad among four plates and top with the fish. Serve.
7. Store any leftovers in an airtight container in the refrigerator for up to 2 days.

**NUTRITION BOOST:** Serve the fish over a bed of lettuce or salad but keep it simple to show off the fish. Add more vegetables on the side, like the Sautéed Lemon Broccoli and Kale (page 132), for a filling meal.

**Per serving:** Calories: 419; Total fat: 24g; Carbohydrates: 17g; Fiber: 5g; Protein: 37g; Calcium: 81mg; Vitamin D: 6mcg; Vitamin $B_{12}$: 2mcg; Iron: 3mg; Zinc: 2mg

# Italian-Style Turkey Meatballs and Zoodles

*Serves 4 / Prep time: 10 minutes / Cook time: 20 minutes*

**GLUTEN-FREE, HIGH-FIBER**

You probably know what zoodles are because this trendy ingredient is in many low-carb recipes. They are spiralized zucchini noodles that take the place of spaghetti or angel hair. Buy zoodles that are already prepared to save time (you can find them in the freezer or produce section). However, if you would like to make them, it's quite easy and something you can do with your kids or with your friends at a group cooking party using a spiralizer. Spiralize one zucchini for each person.

**1 pound ground turkey**

**¼ cup minced onion**

**4 tablespoons pitted olives** (optional)

**1 teaspoon dried oregano**

**1 teaspoon dried thyme**

**1 teaspoon ground fennel**

**½ teaspoon kosher salt**

**1 recipe Basic Marinara** (page 166) **or store-bought**

**8 cups zoodles**

**Fresh chopped parsley, for garnish**

1. Preheat the oven to 375°F. Line a baking sheet with parchment paper.
2. In a large bowl, combine the turkey, onion, olives, oregano, thyme, fennel, and salt until well mixed. Shape the mixture into 1½-inch meatballs and place them on the prepared baking sheet. Bake for 15 to 20 minutes until the internal temperature of the meatballs reaches 160°F.
3. Meanwhile, heat the marinara sauce in a large saucepan over medium heat. Keep the sauce warm until the meatballs are finished cooking.
4. Transfer the meatballs to the sauce and stir to coat.
5. Place 2 cups of zoodles on each plate and top with the marinara sauce and meatballs. Garnish with parsley and serve.
6. Store any leftovers in an airtight container in the refrigerator for up to 4 days.

**VARIATION:** You can use 2 ounces of whole-wheat noodles in place of the zoodles.

**Per serving:** Calories: 489; Total fat: 29g; Carbohydrates: 32g; Fiber: 10g; Protein: 25g; Calcium: 103mg; Vitamin D: <1mcg; Vitamin $B_{12}$: 1mcg; Iron: 5mg; Zinc: 3mg

# Ribboned Squash with Bacon

*Serves 4 / Prep time: 15 minutes / Cook time: 10 minutes*

**GLUTEN-FREE, HIGH-FIBER**

Bacon is not something you need to cut to eat healthfully. This recipe demonstrates how to enjoy bacon in moderation. A single slice of bacon per serving enhances the buttery flavor of the walnuts and sweetness of the squash ribbons. Make the recipe more heart-friendly by omitting the bacon, or vegetarian by swapping out the bacon for cheese or chopped seitan.

**¼ cup dried currants or golden raisins**

**¼ cup red wine vinegar**

**1 pound butternut squash, seeded and skin removed**

**4 bacon slices**

**2 tablespoons extra-virgin olive oil** (optional)

**½ cup chopped, toasted walnuts**

**4 cups arugula**

**Freshly ground black pepper**

**½ cup chopped fresh parsley**

1. In a small bowl, combine the currants and vinegar and allow to soak until tender, about 10 minutes.
2. Using a vegetable peeler, peel the squash into long ribbons into a large bowl. Set aside.
3. Place the bacon slices in a medium skillet over medium heat, cover, and fry for 8 to 10 minutes until cooked through and crispy. Remove the bacon from the heat and drain it on a paper towel. Chop the bacon into bite-size pieces when it's cool enough to handle.
4. Return the pan to medium heat with the bacon fat (or wipe it out and then add the extra-virgin olive oil). Add the walnuts. Heat the walnuts for 2 minutes, then transfer the mixture from the skillet to the squash noodles and toss well. Add the currants with their soaking liquid, along with the arugula and reserved bacon.
5. Season with pepper and serve topped with parsley.
6. Store any leftovers in an airtight container in the refrigerator for up to 4 days.

**VARIATION:** Mix this simple recipe up with other types of nuts or seeds like almonds, pecans, or pumpkin seeds.

**Per serving:** Calories: 272; Total fat: 19g; Carbohydrates: 21g; Fiber: 5g; Protein: 7g; Calcium: 106mg; Vitamin D: 0mcg; Vitamin $B_{12}$: <1mcg; Iron: 2mg; Zinc: 1mg

# Chicken Khao Sen with Rice Noodles

*Serves 2 / Prep time: 5 to 10 minutes / Cook time: 15 minutes*

**GLUTEN-FREE, HIGH-FIBER**

There is a very large Laotian immigrant population in my hometown, and our local cuisine has become all the better as a result. This recipe for Khao Sen is humbly dedicated to this vibrant slice of the culinary community. Red curry paste and fish sauce can be found in the international or Asian foods aisle. If available, Thai basil and Chinese broccoli will give it an even more authentic flavor.

**4 ounces rice noodles**

**2 tablespoons Thai red curry paste**

**½ tablespoon fish sauce** (optional)

**1½ tablespoons extra-virgin olive oil, divided**

**½ pound ground chicken**

**1 head broccoli, ends trimmed**

**½ cup Pickled Red Onions** (page 171)

**1 bunch radishes, cut into matchsticks**

**1 cup bean sprouts**

**1 tablespoon basil, torn**

**1 lime, cut into wedges** (optional)

1. Bring a large saucepan of water to a boil and cook the rice noodles according to the package instructions. Rinse well and allow to cool.
2. Heat the curry paste, fish sauce (if using), and 1 tablespoon of extra-virgin olive oil in a large skillet over medium-high heat. Add the ground chicken and cook thoroughly, about 7 minutes. Set aside in a bowl.
3. Wipe out the skillet and add the remaining ½ tablespoon of extra-virgin olive oil. Add the broccoli and cook until tender, about 3 minutes.
4. Assemble two bowls with the noodles on the bottom and top them with the pickled red onions, cooked chicken, broccoli, radishes, bean sprouts, basil, and a lime wedge (if using, squeeze atop the dish before eating). Serve.
5. Store any leftovers in an airtight container in the refrigerator for up to 4 days.

**VARIATION:** You can replace the rice noodles in this dish with 1 to 2 cups of zoodles (homemade or store-bought) if you're wanting to reduce total carbs in the dish.

**Per serving:** Calories: 615; Total fat: 21g; Carbohydrates: 76g; Fiber: 11g; Protein: 34g; Calcium: 182mg; Vitamin D: 0mcg; Vitamin $B_{12}$: 1mcg; Iron: 4mg; Zinc: 4mg

# Lebanese-Inspired Beef Kebabs with Pickled Onions

*Serves 4 / Prep time: 20 minutes / Cook time: 10 minutes*

GLUTEN-FREE

These spiced beef kebabs are both flavorful and healthy. Using a variety of spices can truly eliminate the need for added salt, which is a bonus for your heart. Serve these tender kebabs with curried rice or throw a corn cob on the grill while you're cooking the beef.

**1 red bell pepper, chopped**

**½ onion, coarsely chopped**

**2 garlic cloves, coarsely chopped**

**1 pound ground beef**

**1½ teaspoons ground cumin**

**1½ teaspoons sumac** (optional)

**1½ teaspoons red pepper flakes**

**1 teaspoon kosher salt**

**Freshly ground black pepper**

**1 tablespoon ice-cold water**

**8 (12-inch) metal skewers (or wooden skewers soaked in warm water for 10 to 30 minutes)**

**1 teaspoon vegetable oil**

**Pickled Red Onions** (page 171)

1. Place the red pepper, onion, and garlic in a food processor and pulse a few times until they're very finely chopped but not pureed. Set aside in a bowl, draining off any excess liquid.

2. Put the beef, processed vegetables, cumin, sumac (if using), red pepper flakes, salt, and a pinch of black pepper into the bowl of a stand mixer with the paddle attached. Work on medium speed until the mix starts sticking to the sides of the bowl, about a minute. Add the ice-cold water and mix for another 5 minutes, until you have a sticky mass. Chill the meat mixture in the freezer for a few minutes or in the refrigerator for at least 30 minutes (or overnight).

3. Divide the meat mixture into 8 balls. With a small bowl of cold water beside you, wet your hands and form the kebab mixture around the skewers, distributing it evenly until you have kofta about 9-by-2-inches thick. Smooth out any holes or tears, then place them on a greaseproof paper–lined baking sheet. (Refrigerate the kofta, covered, if you're not cooking them right away.)

4. Grease a grill pan with the vegetable oil and place it over high heat. Once the pan is hot, grill the kofta until charred on the outside and just cooked through (adjust the heat as necessary), 8 to 10 minutes. Put the grilled kebabs directly on top of the pickled red onions on a platter or individual plates, so the juices drip onto the onions, and serve immediately.

**INGREDIENT TIP:** Try Aleppo pepper flakes instead of red pepper flakes; they're more authentic to the dish and are available in Middle Eastern grocery stores.

**Per serving:** Calories: 321; Total fat: 18g; Carbohydrates: 9g; Fiber: 2g; Protein: 31g; Calcium: 49mg; Vitamin D: <1mcg; Vitamin $B_{12}$: 3mcg; Iron: 4mg; Zinc: 8mg

# Salmon en Papillote

*Serves 2 / Prep time: 15 minutes / Cook time: 15 minutes*

GLUTEN-FREE, HIGH-FIBER

Feeling fancy? En papillote is just French for "baked in paper," a cooking technique that keeps the fish moist and tender. This dish is elegant, delicious, and makes for a fun date-night meal with your sweetheart. You can also use foil instead of parchment and crimp the edges to form a sealed packet.

### FOR THE ROASTED VEGETABLES

**½ pound fresh green beans, trimmed**

**½ onion, cut into ¼-inch-thick slices**

**1 tablespoon extra-virgin olive oil**

**1 teaspoon capers** (optional)

### FOR THE SALMON

**2 teaspoons extra-virgin olive oil, divided**

**2 medium parsnips, cut into ¼-inch-thick rounds, divided**

**2 (4-ounce) salmon fillets**

**2 garlic cloves, thinly sliced, divided**

**1 lemon, divided (½ cut into slices, the other ½ cut into 2 wedges)**

**1 tablespoon chopped fresh thyme, divided**

**Kosher salt**

**Freshly ground black pepper**

### TO MAKE THE ROASTED VEGETABLES

1. Preheat the oven to 400°F. Line a baking sheet with parchment paper.
2. In a medium bowl, toss the green beans, onion, extra-virgin olive oil, and capers (if using) until well coated.
3. Spread the vegetables on half of the baking sheet and set aside until the salmon is ready to bake.

### TO MAKE THE SALMON

4. Cut two pieces of parchment paper, fold them in half, and cut each into a heart shape (about 10 to 12 inches in circumference). Lightly brush the parchment with ½ teaspoon of extra-virgin olive oil.

5. Open one of the hearts and place half the parsnips on the right half in the center, fanning them out. Place one piece of salmon on the fanned parsnips. Add half the garlic, half the lemon slices, half the thyme, ½ teaspoon of extra-virgin olive oil, and a pinch each of kosher salt and pepper.

6. Seal the packet by folding the left half of the heart over the right side. Fold along the edge of the heart and create a seal. Repeat with the other piece of parchment.

7. Place the packets on the empty side of the baking sheet and bake until the salmon is cooked through, 10 to 15 minutes. Allow the fish to rest a few minutes before serving with the roasted green beans and remaining lemon wedges.

8. Store any leftovers in an airtight container in the refrigerator for 1 to 2 days.

**VARIATION:** There are many possibilities for spices and herbs to use with salmon. Favorites of mine include tarragon, thyme, and lemon. If I'm lucky enough to have lavender, I'll add some of that, too. Very French!

---

**Per serving:** Calories: 378; Total fat: 19g; Carbohydrates: 31g; Fiber: 9g; Protein: 26g; Calcium: 104mg; Vitamin D: 12mcg; Vitamin $B_{12}$: 0mcg; Iron: 3mg; Zinc: 1mg

# Cherry Barbecue Chicken Cutlets

*Serves 4 / Prep time: 10 minutes / Cook time: 5 minutes*

**5-INGREDIENT, GLUTEN-FREE**

Chicken remains undefeated as the go-to dinner protein. Boneless, skinless chicken cutlets are the fastest to cook, but if you have more time, you can also use other cuts of chicken. Many supermarkets carry chicken cutlets, but you can also prepare your own. Carefully cut the chicken breasts horizontally in half and pound them to a quarter-inch thickness between sheets of plastic wrap to reduce any mess. Consider serving these with Avocado Slaw (page 142) or Sautéed Lemon Broccoli and Kale (page 132) on the side.

**1½ pounds boneless, skinless chicken cutlets**

**1 recipe Cherry Barbecue Sauce** (page 165) **or store-bought, divided**

**1½ tablespoons extra-virgin olive oil**

### STOVETOP METHOD

1. Marinate the chicken in half the barbecue sauce in the refrigerator for up to 1 day.
2. The following day, heat the extra-virgin olive oil in a large skillet over high heat. Add the cutlets and cook without disturbing them. Make sure they do not touch, about 1 to 2 inches apart. Cook until brown, 2 to 3 minutes. Flip, and cook another 30 seconds.
3. Repeat with the remaining chicken cutlets if they do not all fit in one pan without overcrowding.
4. Allow the chicken to rest for 5 minutes before serving.
5. Meanwhile, heat the remaining sauce in a small saucepan, then serve with the cooked chicken.

### GRILL METHOD

1. Marinate the chicken in half the barbecue sauce in the refrigerator for up to 1 day.
2. Remove the chicken from the marinade and place it on a plate, removing any excess sauce. Discard the marinade.
3. Place the remaining sauce in a small saucepan over low heat until warm.
4. Prepare the grill grates and heat them to between 425°F and 450°F.
5. When the grill is hot, lightly oil the cooking grate, arrange the cutlets about 2 inches apart, and cook for 2 to 3 minutes. Turn the cutlets over and grill until cooked through, about 30 seconds more.
6. Let the grilled cutlets rest for 5 minutes before serving them with the remaining warm sauce. Store any leftovers in an airtight container in the refrigerator for 1 to 2 days.

**MAKE IT EASIER:** If you have a favorite barbecue sauce, go ahead and use it, but check the nutrition label. Most store-bought barbecue sauces are quite high in carbohydrates, sugar, and sodium.

---

**Per serving:** Calories: 272; Total fat: 6g; Carbohydrates: 16g; Fiber: 3g; Protein: 40g; Calcium: 36mg; Vitamin D: 0mcg; Vitamin $B_{12}$: 0mcg; Iron: 1mg; Zinc: <1mg

# Miso Skirt Steak

*Serves 4 / Prep time: 20 minutes / Cook time: 5 to 10 minutes*

I promised you in the introduction that you would see a few favorites and, yes, that means this perfectly prepared steak. Red meat can fit into a healthy diet, as long as it's in moderation and your focus is still on whole, plant-based foods. While meat shouldn't be the primary source of your calories or macronutrients, know that you can still enjoy steak on occasion. Here it is, flavorfully prepared with miso and soy.

**3 tablespoons yellow miso**

**1 tablespoon low-sodium soy sauce or tamari**

**½ tablespoon sesame oil**

**2 tablespoons chile-garlic sauce**

**1½ pounds skirt steak, patted dry**

**3 tablespoons rice vinegar**

**1 tablespoon vegetable oil, divided**

1. In a medium bowl, whisk together the miso, soy sauce, sesame oil, and chile-garlic sauce. Put 1 tablespoon of the sauce in a separate small bowl and set aside. Place the steak in the bowl with the remaining sauce and marinate it at room temperature for 10 to 15 minutes.
2. Stir the vinegar and ½ tablespoon of vegetable oil into the reserved sauce and set aside.
3. Remove the steak from the bowl and pat it dry.
4. Heat the remaining ½ tablespoon of vegetable oil in a large skillet over medium-high heat, add the steak, and cook without disturbing it. Cook for 2 to 3 minutes, until brown. Flip the steak and repeat with the other side (bring to 125°F internal temperature for medium rare and 135°F for medium). Transfer the steak to a plate, tent it with foil, and allow it to rest for 5 to 10 minutes.
5. Serve with the sauce on the side.

**NUTRIENT BOOST:** Keep the meal simple and serve the steak with salad greens, cooked whole grains, Cauliflower Rice (page 138), or a mixture of all three options.

**Per serving:** Calories: 478; Total fat: 36g; Carbohydrates: 4g; Fiber: 1g; Protein: 32g; Calcium: 10mg; Vitamin D: 0mcg; Vitamin $B_{12}$: <1mcg; Iron: 3mg; Zinc: <1mg

# Herbed Buttermilk Chicken

*Serves 4 / Prep time: 5 minutes / Cook time: 25 minutes*

GLUTEN-FREE, ONE PAN

The chicken in this exceptional dish needs to be marinated in the buttermilk seasoning (brine), so you will need to plan ahead when you make it, but it cooks quite quickly after that. Marinating will not only help tenderize your bird, but it will also give the poultry a deep, rich flavor. Try serving this with Herbed Tomato Salad (page 56) to round out the meal.

**1½ pounds boneless, skinless chicken breasts**

**4 cups buttermilk**

**Pinch kosher salt**

**Pinch freshly ground black pepper**

**1 cup thinly sliced yellow onion**

**2 tablespoons canola oil**

**¼ cup Italian seasoning**

**1 lemon, cut into wedges**

1. In a large bowl or sealable plastic bag, combine the chicken, buttermilk, salt, and pepper. Cover or seal and refrigerate for at least 1 hour and up to 24 hours.
2. When the chicken is ready to cook, preheat the oven to 425°F. Line a baking sheet with parchment paper.
3. Remove the chicken from the buttermilk brine and pat it dry. Place the chicken on the prepared baking sheet along with the onion, and drizzle everything with the canola oil. Toss together on the baking sheet (this will save you a bowl) to coat the chicken and onion evenly.
4. Bake for 25 minutes or until the chicken is cooked through. (If the chicken is thick, you can cut the breasts in half lengthwise. It will cut down on your cook time by half or less. Check the chicken after it's cooked for 8 minutes if the breasts are thin.)
5. Allow the chicken to rest and sprinkle it and the onions with the Italian seasoning.
6. Serve with a squeeze of lemon juice.

**INGREDIENT TIP:** If you don't have Italian seasoning at home, it can be substituted with a combination of thyme, oregano, parsley, basil, or marjoram. Use a blend of whichever you have on hand. You can also use the Middle Eastern spice blend za'atar with this recipe.

**Per serving:** Calories: 437; Total fat: 20g; Carbohydrates: 19g; Fiber: 2g; Protein: 46g; Calcium: 352mg; Vitamin D: 3mcg; Vitamin $B_{12}$: 1mcg; Iron: 3mg; Zinc: 1mg

# Chicken Sausage and Cauliflower Pizza

*Serves 2 to 4 / Prep time: 5 minutes / Cook time: 10 minutes*

**5-INGREDIENT, GLUTEN-FREE, ONE PAN**

As little as five years ago, you would have had to make your own cauliflower pizza crust because this product was not on the culinary radar. Now even small grocery stores carry cauliflower pizza crust as a substitute for wheat-based crusts. If you prefer, you can use pita, naan, or sliced vegetables (eggplant or zucchini, for example) as the pizza base instead of the store-bought crust with delicious results.

**1 store-bought cauliflower pizza crust, thawed**

**¼ cup Basic Marinara** (page 166) **or store-bought**

**1 link cooked chicken sausage, casing removed, sliced**

**1 red bell pepper, diced**

**2 ounces shredded mozzarella cheese**

1. Preheat the oven according to the cauliflower pizza crust's package instructions.
2. Place the cauliflower crust on a baking sheet and spread it evenly with the marinara sauce. Evenly distribute the chicken sausage, bell pepper, and mozzarella cheese on the pizza.
3. Bake the pizza according to instructions, usually 7 to 10 minutes if baked at 425°F.
4. Slice and serve.
5. Store any leftovers in an airtight container in the refrigerator for 3 to 4 days.

**VARIATION:** The options for pizza toppings are endless. Add any vegetables—like small broccoli florets, cooked mushrooms, diced onions, olives, canned artichokes, fresh tomatoes, fresh herbs, or even salad greens—to the sauce-covered crust and bake.

**Per serving:** Calories: 408; Total fat: 16g; Carbohydrates: 49g; Fiber: 3g; Protein: 15g; Calcium: 203mg; Vitamin D: <1mcg; Vitamin $B_{12}$: <1mcg; Iron: 1mg; Zinc: 1mg

# Turkey Bolognese with Chickpea Pasta

*Serves 4 / Prep time: 5 minutes / Cook time: 25 minutes*

**GLUTEN-FREE, HIGH-FIBER**

Making traditional Bolognese sauce is a long and arduous process. The classic Italian dish made with pork and beef can take all day. But I've come up with a recipe that is much faster and has fewer carbs. Chickpea pasta is a tasty alternative to wheat-based pasta with fewer carbohydrates and more protein and fiber, so it leaves your tummy fuller for longer. Preparing the vegetables for the sauce in a food processor cuts down on time considerably.

**1 onion, coarsely chopped**

**1 large carrot, coarsely chopped**

**2 celery stalks, coarsely chopped**

**1 tablespoon extra-virgin olive oil**

**1 pound ground turkey**

**½ cup milk**

**¾ cup red or white wine**

**1 (28-ounce) can diced tomatoes**

**10 ounces cooked chickpea pasta**

1. Place the onion, carrots, and celery in a food processor and pulse until finely chopped.
2. Heat the extra-virgin olive oil in a Dutch oven or medium skillet over medium-high heat. Sauté the chopped vegetables for 3 to 5 minutes, or until softened. Add the ground turkey, breaking the poultry into smaller pieces, and cook for 5 minutes.
3. Add the milk and wine and cook until the liquid is nearly evaporated (turn up the heat to high to quicken the process).
4. Add the tomatoes and bring the sauce to a simmer. Reduce the heat to low and simmer for 10 to 15 minutes.
5. Meanwhile, cook the pasta according to the package instructions and set aside.
6. Serve the sauce with the cooked chickpea pasta.
7. Store any leftovers in an airtight container in the refrigerator for 3 to 4 days.

**Per serving:** Calories: 601; Total fat: 23g; Carbohydrates: 58g; Fiber: 11g; Protein: 39g; Calcium: 146mg; Vitamin D: 1mcg; Vitamin $B_{12}$: 2mcg; Iron: 7mg; Zinc: 3mg

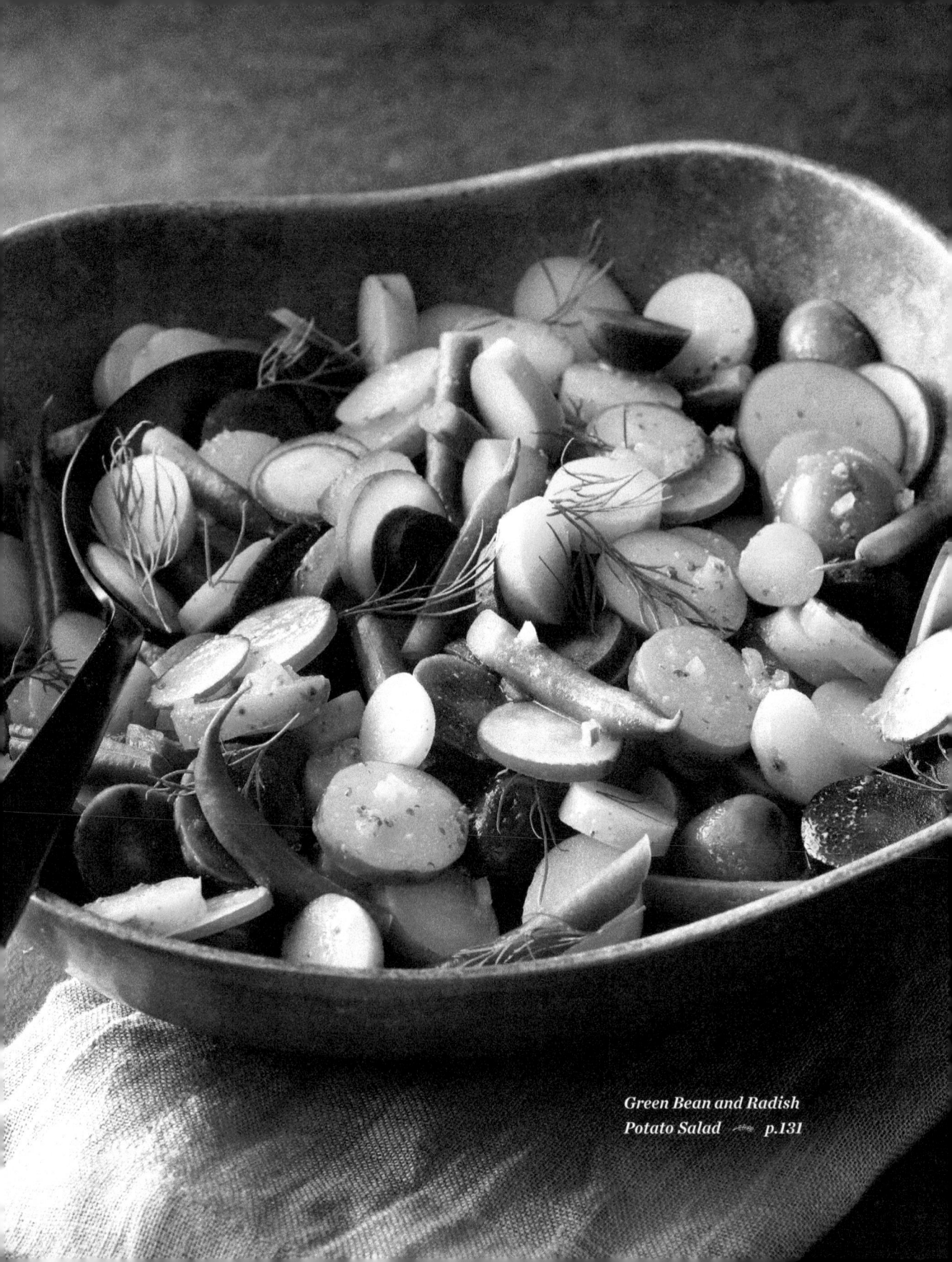

*Green Bean and Radish Potato Salad* p.131

CHAPTER SEVEN

# Sides and Snacks

Sides and snacks are often treated as an afterthought, not given the same consideration as large-plate main courses, or dessert. But 33 percent of Americans snack at least once per day (according to a 2019 survey from the International Food Information Council), and some statistics have that number as high as 94 percent (Mintel, 2015). Similarly, a supplementary side dish with your main course is also a common feature of dining. We tackle small plates in this chapter and take particular care because the "extras" like snacks and sides can be one of the most important factors when trying to cut back on carbs. You'll recognize some classics here, as well as variations on those classics. For example, kale chip nachos are a surprisingly satisfying alternative to the traditional corn tortilla chip dish. When trying to keep yourself satisfied throughout the day, this could be the most crucial section of the book.

Cucumber Roll-Ups ..... 125

Eggplant Pizzas ..... 126

Roasted Carrot and Chickpea Dip ..... 127

Kale Chip Nachos ..... 128

Lemony White Bean Puree ..... 130

Green Bean and Radish Potato Salad ..... 131

Sautéed Lemon Broccoli and Kale ..... 132

Roasted Asparagus with Romesco Sauce ..... 133

Charred Sesame Broccoli ..... 135

Smashed Cucumber Salad ..... 136

Garlic Roasted Radishes ..... 137

Cauliflower Rice ..... 138

Cajun-Style Collards ..... 139

Mashed Sweet Potatoes ..... 140

Charred Miso Cabbage ..... 141

Avocado Slaw ..... 142

# Cucumber Roll-Ups

*Serves 2 to 4 / Prep time: 5 minutes*

**5-INGREDIENT, GLUTEN-FREE, NO-COOK, ONE BOWL, VEGETARIAN**

Roll-ups are easy to make and ideal for a grab-and-go snack. Use any wrap you'd like for this recipe and read your labels to ensure the carbs are within your personal limit. Some of my favorite wraps are the raw vegetable versions (cauliflower, kale, tomato) or those with a base of almond flour, coconut, corn, whole wheat (lavash), or potato lefse.

**2 (6-inch) gluten-free wraps**
**2 tablespoons cream cheese**
**1 medium cucumber, cut into long strips**
**2 tablespoons fresh mint**

1. Place the wraps on your work surface and spread them evenly with the cream cheese. Top with the cucumber and mint.
2. Roll the wraps up from one side to the other, kind of like a burrito. Slice into 1-inch bites or keep whole.
3. Serve.
4. Store any leftovers in an airtight container in the refrigerator for 1 to 2 days.

**MAKE IT EASIER:** Depending on the flexibility of the wrap you've chosen, rolling this snack can be challenging. If the product is stiff, try microwaving it for a few seconds to soften it or warming it in a dry skillet over low heat.

**Per serving:** Calories: 168; Total fat: 8g; Carbohydrates: 21g; Fiber: 3g; Protein: 5g; Calcium: 35mg; Vitamin D: 0mcg; Vitamin $B_{12}$: <1mcg; Iron: <1mg; Zinc: <1mg

# Eggplant Pizzas

*Serves 4 to 6 / Prep time: 5 minutes / Cook time: 15 minutes*

GLUTEN-FREE, HIGH-FIBER, VEGETARIAN

There was a story once of a young boy who simply *hated* eggplant, and couldn't stand the sight of this vegetable. What did his mother do to ensure he was getting the fiber, potassium, and the B vitamins found in this nightshade? Turn it into pizza, of course. You're sure to enjoy this light pizza and extra serving of vegetables, too.

**2 pounds eggplant, cut into ½-inch-thick slices**

**2 tablespoons extra-virgin olive oil**

**Kosher salt**

**Freshly ground black pepper**

**1 cup Basic Marinara** (page 166) **or store-bought**

**1 cup crushed tomatoes**

**½ onion, thinly sliced**

**1 cup sliced mushrooms**

**1½ cups shredded mozzarella cheese**

1. Preheat the oven to 425°F. Line a baking sheet with parchment paper.
2. Brush both sides of the eggplant slices with extra-virgin olive oil and lightly season them with salt and pepper. Place the slices on the prepared baking sheet and bake until the top side of the eggplant browns, about 7 minutes.
3. Meanwhile, in a small bowl, stir together the marinara and crushed tomatoes until combined.
4. When the eggplant is browned, turn the slices over. Top them with marinara followed by the onions and mushrooms. Sprinkle with the cheese and bake until the cheese melts, 5 to 8 minutes.
5. Serve immediately.
6. Store any leftovers in an airtight container in the refrigerator for 3 to 4 days.

**MAKE IT EASIER:** You can also use a toaster oven to make this tempting snack. It will heat the pizzas much faster and easier if you have one on hand.

**Per serving:** Calories: 268; Total fat: 15g; Carbohydrates: 24g; Fiber: 9g; Protein: 12g; Calcium: 257mg; Vitamin D: <1mcg; Vitamin $B_{12}$: <1mcg; Iron: 1mg; Zinc: 2mg

# Roasted Carrot and Chickpea Dip

*Makes 3 cups / Prep time: 10 minutes / Cook time: 15 minutes*

GLUTEN-FREE, VEGETARIAN

Dips are often crowd favorites at parties because you don't just get to sample the dip itself, you also enjoy an assortment of "dippers." It is like having two snacks in one! This sweet and spicy dip is ideal for a group, but it is just as good when you're looking for your own snack. It keeps well, so make it in advance to have on hand when you're feeling hungry.

**4 medium carrots, quartered lengthwise**

**¼ cup plus 2 teaspoons extra-virgin olive oil, divided**

**Pinch kosher salt**

**Pinch freshly ground black pepper**

**1 (15-ounce) can chickpeas, drained and rinsed**

**1 garlic clove, minced**

**1 red chile** (optional)

**Zest and juice of 1 lemon**

**2 tablespoons tahini**

**1 tablespoon Harissa** (page 169)

**½ teaspoon ground cumin**

**¼ teaspoon ground coriander**

**Pomegranate arils (seeds)** (optional)

**Cilantro, chopped** (optional)

1. Preheat the oven to 425°F. Line a baking sheet with parchment paper.
2. In a medium bowl, toss the carrots with 2 teaspoons of extra-virgin olive oil, the salt, and the pepper. Spread them in a single layer on the prepared baking sheet and roast until tender, about 15 minutes. Turn the carrots over halfway through.
3. Meanwhile, place the chickpeas, garlic, chile, lemon zest and juice, tahini, harissa, cumin, and coriander in a food processor. Set aside. Add the carrots to the processor when they are cooked. Pulse until the mixture is coarse. Scrape the bowl down, then turn the processor back on while you drizzle the remaining ¼ cup of extra-virgin olive oil through the feed tube of the machine. Adjust the seasonings as desired. If it's too thick, add water to thin.
4. Top with pomegranate seeds and chopped cilantro (if using,) and Serve with cut vegetables.
5. Store any leftovers in an airtight container in the refrigerator for up to 4 days.

**SUBSTITUTION TIP:** Use tomato paste instead of harissa if you don't have it ready, or if you want less spice.

**Per ¼-cup serving:** Calories: 105; Total fat: 7g; Carbohydrates: 8g; Fiber: 2g; Protein: 2g; Calcium: 29mg; Vitamin D: 0mcg; Vitamin $B_{12}$: 0mcg; Iron: 1mg; Zinc: <1mg

# Kale Chip Nachos

*Serves 2 to 4 / Prep time: 10 minutes / Cook time: 20 minutes*

GLUTEN-FREE, HIGH-FIBER, VEGETARIAN

Kale was everywhere for a while, a "superfood" that seemed to descend into a parody considering its appearance in so many different products and recipes. But, as it turns out, there was something to the hype after all. And when you're looking for something to snack on while watching the game or your favorite show, you want to make sure it's something that isn't going to do too much damage to your body in the long run. This version of nachos uses kale as the base, so you can snack away while getting the nutritional boost that comes from this hearty green alongside sweet potato and black beans.

**1 bunch kale, torn into bite-size pieces**

**3 tablespoons extra-virgin olive oil, divided**

**2 teaspoons ground cumin, divided**

**1 large sweet potato, cut into ¼-inch-thick rounds**

**1 (15-ounce) can black beans, rinsed and drained**

**½ teaspoon ground coriander**

**1 teaspoon chili powder**

OPTIONAL TOPPINGS

**Avocado slices**

**Salsa**

**Jicama, sliced**

**Red onion, sliced**

**Fresh cilantro**

**Fresh chiles, minced**

**Fresh tomatoes, diced**

1. Preheat the oven to 225°F. Line a baking sheet with parchment paper.
2. In a large bowl, toss the kale with 1 tablespoon of oil and 1 teaspoon of cumin. Use your hands to massage the kale and evenly distribute the oil.
3. Spread the kale in a single even layer on the prepared baking sheet. (You may need two lined baking sheets for this.) Bake for 15 minutes, then flip and toss, and bake for another 5 to 10 minutes.
4. Meanwhile, heat 1 tablespoon of oil in a large skillet over medium-high heat. Arrange the sweet potato rounds in a single layer in the skillet, cover, and let them cook until they begin to brown on the bottom, about 3 minutes. Flip the potatoes over and cook for 3 to 5 minutes more.

5. Add the black beans to the skillet with the remaining 1 tablespoon of oil, remaining 1 teaspoon of cumin, the coriander, and chili powder. Cook for 3 minutes, then set aside and keep warm if the kale is not yet finished baking.
6. Serve on a platter, starting with the kale as a base, topped with sweet potatoes, black beans, and finally, any optional toppings.
7. Store any leftovers in an airtight container in the refrigerator for 3 to 4 days.

**VARIATION:** You can use any kind of canned beans or lentils in place of the black beans for additional variety with this recipe.

**Per serving:** Calories: 504; Total fat: 23g; Carbohydrates: 63g; Fiber: 21g; Protein: 16g; Calcium: 266mg; Vitamin D: 0mcg; Vitamin $B_{12}$: 0mcg; Iron: 7mg; Zinc: 2mg

# Lemony White Bean Puree

*Makes ~2 cups / Prep time: 10 minutes*

**GLUTEN-FREE, HIGH-FIBER, NO-COOK, VEGETARIAN**

This recipe calls for herbs de Provence, an essential herb blend native to the southern region of France. You may see it appear in other Mediterranean cuisines. It adds a distinct flavor to dishes like chicken, roasted vegetables, and grilled fish. There are many variations of the herb blend, but you will usually find basil, fennel, marjoram, parsley, rosemary, tarragon, and thyme. Some blends include lavender as well.

**1 (15-ounce) can white beans, drained and rinsed**

**1 small onion, coarsely chopped**

**1 garlic clove, minced**

**Zest and juice of 1 lemon**

**½ teaspoon herbs de Provence**

**3 tablespoons extra-virgin olive oil, divided**

**1 tablespoon chopped fresh parsley**

1. Place the beans, onion, garlic, lemon zest and juice, and herbs in a food processor and pulse until smooth. While the machine is running, slowly stream in 2 tablespoons of extra-virgin olive oil. If the mixture is too thick, add water very slowly until you've reached the desired consistency.
2. Transfer the puree to a medium serving bowl. Top with the remaining 1 tablespoon of extra-virgin olive oil and the parsley.
3. Serve with your favorite vegetable or flatbread of choice. Store any leftovers in an airtight container in the refrigerator for up to 4 days.

**VARIATION:** Other dried herbs can be substituted for herbs de Provence. Choose one or more of the dried herbs listed on pages 23 and 24 and alter the dip to your liking.

**Per ½-cup serving:** Calories: 197; Total fat: 11g; Carbohydrates: 21g; Fiber: 6g; Protein: 6g; Calcium: 78mg; Vitamin D: 0mcg; Vitamin $B_{12}$: 0mcg; Iron: 2mg; Zinc: <1mg

# Green Bean and Radish Potato Salad

*Serves 6 / Prep time: 10 minutes / Cook time: 20 minutes*

**GLUTEN-FREE, ONE POT, VEGETARIAN**

Fingerling potatoes, those small multicolored potatoes similar in size to fingers (hence their name), have a robust, earthy, and buttery flavor. They are wonderful in salads because they keep their shape after cooking due to their firmness. If you cannot find fingerlings, Yukon Gold potatoes will also work in this recipe.

**Kosher salt**

**6 ounces fresh green beans, trimmed and cut into 1-inch pieces**

**1½ pounds fingerling potatoes**

**⅓ cup extra-virgin olive oil**

**2 tablespoons freshly squeezed lemon juice**

**1 tablespoon Dijon or whole-grain mustard**

**1 shallot, minced**

**8 radishes, thinly sliced**

**¼ cup fresh dill, chopped**

**Freshly ground black pepper**

1. Place a small saucepan filled three-quarters full of water and a pinch of salt over high heat and bring it to a boil. Add the green beans and boil for 2 minutes, then transfer them with a slotted spoon to a colander. Run the beans under cold running water until cool and transfer to a medium bowl.
2. Place the potatoes in the same pot of boiling water, reduce the heat to low, and simmer until tender, about 12 minutes.
3. Meanwhile, combine the extra-virgin olive oil, lemon juice, mustard, and shallot in a jar. Seal with the lid and shake vigorously. If you don't have a jar with a fitted lid, you can also whisk the ingredients in a bowl.
4. Transfer the cooked potatoes to a colander and cool them under cold running water. When they're cool enough to handle, slice the potatoes into thin rounds.
5. Add the potatoes and dressing to the bowl with the green beans, along with the radishes and dill, and toss to combine.
6. Season with salt and pepper and serve.
7. Store any leftovers in an airtight container in the refrigerator for 3 to 4 days.

**Per serving:** Calories: 208; Total fat: 12g; Carbohydrates: 24g; Fiber: 3g; Protein: 3g; Calcium: 33mg; Vitamin D: 0mcg; Vitamin $B_{12}$: 0mcg; Iron: 3mg; Zinc: <1mg

# Sautéed Lemon Broccoli and Kale

*Serves 4 to 6 / Prep time: 5 minutes / Cook time: 15 minutes*

**GLUTEN-FREE, HIGH-FIBER, VEGETARIAN**

This dish celebrates green vegetables—something parents have struggled to get their children to eat for decades. It is simple dishes like this one that remind us that green vegetables can be just as flavorful as anything that comes from an animal. Cumin seeds, which make everything better, garlic, and a punch of flavor from fresh lemon should convince even the most skeptical of diners to eat their greens.

**1 large head broccoli, cut into small florets**

**2 tablespoons extra-virgin olive oil**

**1 bunch kale, torn into 1- to 2-inch pieces**

**2 garlic cloves, minced**

**½ teaspoon cumin seeds**

**1 lemon, cut into wedges**

1. Bring a medium saucepan filled three-quarters full of water to a boil over high heat. Add the broccoli and boil for 3 minutes. Drain the broccoli and run it under cold water until completely cool.
2. Heat the extra-virgin olive oil in a large skillet over medium-high heat. Add the broccoli, kale, garlic, and cumin and sauté for 2 to 3 minutes. Remove the skillet from the heat and serve with freshly squeezed lemon.
3. Store any leftovers in an airtight container in the refrigerator for 3 to 4 days.

**VARIATION:** Add other citrus or herbs to boost the flavor profile of the dish. Toss in red pepper flakes while you're at it for a touch of heat. This side pairs beautifully with any protein-heavy entrée like Miso Skirt Steak (page 118).

**Per serving:** Calories: 126; Total fat: 8g; Carbohydrates: 13g; Fiber: 5g; Protein: 5g; Calcium: 134mg; Vitamin D: 0mcg; Vitamin $B_{12}$: 0mcg; Iron: 2mg; Zinc: 1mg

# Roasted Asparagus with Romesco Sauce

*Serves 2 to 4 / Prep time: 5 minutes / Cook time: 15 minutes*

**5-INGREDIENT, HIGH-FIBER, VEGETARIAN**

Asparagus is one of the true harbingers of warm weather, along with the birdsongs and delicate budding flowers, of course. The moment fresh asparagus becomes available, try this lovely side dish to celebrate the season. The Romesco Sauce found on page 170 brings out the natural, earthy flavor of the asparagus and adds a punch of its own to create a perfect balance. You can roast or grill the asparagus—both are equally tasty.

**1 bunch asparagus, woody ends removed**

**1 tablespoon extra-virgin olive oil**

**¼ to ½ cup Romesco Sauce** (page 170) **or store-bought**

## ROASTED METHOD

1. Preheat the oven to 425°F. Line a baking sheet with parchment paper.
2. In a medium bowl, toss the asparagus with the extra-virgin olive oil.
3. Place the asparagus on the baking sheet and roast until tender, 12 to 15 minutes.
4. Remove the asparagus from the heat, arrange it on a serving platter, top it with romesco sauce, and serve.

continued

### GRILL METHOD

1. Preheat the grill to high heat.
2. In a medium bowl, toss the asparagus with the extra-virgin olive oil.
3. Place the asparagus on a grill pan or directly on the grill grates and sear for 2 to 4 minutes until tender, turning them as often as you need to avoid burning.
4. Remove the asparagus from the heat, arrange it on a serving platter, top it with romesco sauce, and serve.
5. Store any leftovers in an airtight container in the refrigerator for 3 to 4 days.

**VARIATION:** Instead of Romesco Sauce, accent the asparagus with citrus by tossing the spears in Lemon Vinaigrette Dressing (page 159). No need to use additional oil, just the asparagus and the dressing work fine.

**Per serving:** Calories: 183; Total fat: 13g; Carbohydrates: 14g; Fiber: 6g; Protein: 7g; Calcium: 80mg; Vitamin D: 0mcg; Vitamin $B_{12}$: 0mcg; Iron: 5mg; Zinc: 2mg

# Charred Sesame Broccoli

*Serves 4 / Prep time: 5 minutes / Cook time: 15 minutes*

**5-INGREDIENT, VEGETARIAN**

Broccoli is ubiquitous, but often people use the same techniques and overcook until it's army green in color and turns to mush. This is highly undesirable in both appearance and flavor. Try cooking your broccoli using this method and you'll have everyone reaching for it. Broccoli is loaded with fiber, calcium, folate, potassium, and iron and supports bone health, brain function, and heart health.

**1 tablespoon extra-virgin olive oil**

**1 tablespoon low-sodium soy sauce**

**½ tablespoon sesame oil**

**1 head broccoli**

**1 tablespoon toasted sesame seeds**

1. Preheat the oven to 450°F. Line a baking sheet with parchment paper.
2. In a medium bowl, whisk together the extra-virgin olive oil, soy sauce, and sesame oil. Add the broccoli and toss to evenly coat it.
3. Spread the coated broccoli on the prepared baking sheet and bake for 10 minutes, until tender.
4. Remove the sheet from the oven, flip the broccoli over, and return it to the oven for an additional 5 to 10 minutes.
5. Serve the broccoli with toasted sesame seeds on top.
6. Store any leftovers in an airtight container in the refrigerator for up to 4 days.

**INGREDIENT TIP:** You can use regular broccoli here, but also give Chinese broccoli a try if it's available. Called *gai lan,* it is one of the most popular greens in all of China and has a stronger, slightly bitter note that lends itself well to the sesame and the soy of this dish. Broccoli rabe is also an inspired choice.

**Per serving:** Calories: 110; Total fat: 7g; Carbohydrates: 11g; Fiber: 4g; Protein: 5g; Calcium: 75mg; Vitamin D: 0mcg; Vitamin $B_{12}$: 0mcg; Iron: 1mg; Zinc: 1mg

# Smashed Cucumber Salad

*Serves 4 to 6 / Prep time: 10 minutes*

**GLUTEN-FREE, NO-COOK, VEGETARIAN**

Smashing cucumbers for a salad is a standard technique in many parts of Asia. Once you've tried it, you'll understand why it's such a great idea, and not just for taking out your aggression. Smashing a cucumber changes the way it picks up the flavors. More cucumber cells open up and allow for some water to escape, while absorbing other added ingredients, thus changing the overall taste.

**2 pounds mini cucumbers (English or Persian), unpeeled**

**½ teaspoon kosher salt**

**1 tablespoon extra-virgin olive oil**

**¾ teaspoon ground cumin**

**¼ teaspoon turmeric**

**Juice of 1 lime**

**½ cup cilantro leaves**

1. Cut the cucumbers crosswise into 4-inch pieces and again in half lengthwise.
2. On a work surface, place one cucumber, flesh-side down. Place the side of the knife blade on the cucumber and carefully smash down lightly with your hand. Alternatively, put in a plastic bag, seal, and smash with a rolling pin or similar tool. Be careful not to break the bag. The skin of the cucumber should crack and flesh will break away. Repeat with all the cucumbers and cut the smashed pieces on a bias into bite-size pieces.
3. Transfer the cucumber pieces to a strainer and toss them with the salt. Allow the cucumbers to rest for at least 15 minutes.
4. Meanwhile, prepare the dressing by whisking together the extra-virgin olive oil, cumin, turmeric, and lime juice in a small bowl.
5. When the cucumbers are ready, shake them to remove any excess liquid. Transfer the cucumbers to a large bowl with the dressing and cilantro and toss to combine. Serve.
6. Store any leftovers in an airtight container in the refrigerator for up to 2 days.

**MAKE IT EASIER:** Use fresh, firm-fleshed cucumbers and avoid those that are older and soft. Your standard greenhouse variety commonly found in grocery stores will work just fine, but I would strongly suggest removing the seeds before smashing them.

**Per serving:** Calories: 69; Total fat: 4g; Carbohydrates: 10g; Fiber: 3g; Protein: 2g; Calcium: 44mg; Vitamin D: 0mcg; Vitamin $B_{12}$: 0mcg; Iron: 1mg; Zinc: 1mg

# Garlic Roasted Radishes

*Serves 2 to 4 / Prep time: 5 minutes / Cook time: 15 minutes*

**5-INGREDIENT, GLUTEN-FREE, VEGETARIAN**

Radishes are one of spring's greatest treats. They are cruciferous, like broccoli and cabbage, which means they have many of the same cancer-fighting compounds as these powerhouse vegetables. They also have a positive impact on the fight against diabetes, as some studies suggest eating radishes may help improve blood sugar control. Radishes are also delicious and come in a multitude of colors that look great on the plate.

**1 pound radishes, halved**
**1 tablespoon canola oil**
**Pinch kosher salt**
**4 garlic cloves, thinly sliced**
**¼ cup chopped fresh dill**

1. Preheat the oven to 425°F. Line a baking sheet with parchment paper.
2. In a medium bowl, toss the radishes with the canola oil and salt. Spread the vegetables on the prepared baking sheet and roast for 10 minutes. Remove the sheet from the oven, add the garlic, mix well, and return to the oven for 5 minutes.
3. Remove the radishes from the oven, adjust the seasoning as desired, and serve topped with dill on a serving plate or as a side dish.
4. Store any leftovers in an airtight container in the refrigerator for 3 to 4 days.

**VARIATION:** This salad can be exceptionally pretty if you use a variety of radishes. Look for watermelon radish, Easter egg, purple ninja, cherriette, or daikon if you want to experiment with colors. If you decide to take this route, cut the radishes to a similar size before roasting, so they cook at the same rate.

**Per serving:** Calories: 105; Total fat: 7g; Carbohydrates: 10g; Fiber: 4g; Protein: 2g; Calcium: 70mg; Vitamin D: 0mcg; Vitamin $B_{12}$: 0mcg; Iron: 1mg; Zinc: 1mg

# Cauliflower Rice

*Makes 2½ cups / Prep time: 5 minutes / Cook time: 5 minutes*

**5-INGREDIENT, GLUTEN-FREE, VEGETARIAN**

Cauliflower rice cooks much faster than regular rice, so it can cut down on the cooking time if you use it in dishes like the Cauli-Lettuce Wraps (page 74) or Tuna Poke with Riced Broccoli (page 105). This side dish is also a wonderful replacement for grains in general, especially when you have other carbohydrates in your meal that could cross over into excessive amounts.

**1½ pounds cauliflower, coarsely chopped**

**½ tablespoon extra-virgin olive oil**

**Kosher salt**

**Freshly ground black pepper**

1. Pulse the cauliflower in a food processor until it has a crumbly texture, almost like rice. Be careful not to over-pulse and make it too fine. It's okay to have some larger chunks. Another option is to use a box grater if you don't have a food processor. Put the crumbled cauliflower in a bowl and set aside.
2. Heat the oil in a large skillet over medium-high heat. Add the cauliflower, coat it with hot oil, and sauté 3 to 5 minutes. Season with salt and pepper and serve.
3. Store any leftovers in an airtight container in the refrigerator for 3 to 4 days.

**VARIATION:** Add any spice blend you want to jazz up the flavor of this rice. Try curry powder or add some fresh cilantro with lime, or fresh parsley with lemon.

**Per ½-cup serving:** Calories: 46; Total fat: 2g; Carbohydrates: 7g; Fiber: 3g; Protein: 3g; Calcium: 30mg; Vitamin D: 0mcg; Vitamin $B_{12}$: 0mcg; Iron: 1mg; Zinc: <1mg

# Cajun-Style Collards

*Serves 4 to 6 / Prep time: 10 minutes / Cook time: 20 minutes*

**GLUTEN-FREE, HIGH-FIBER, ONE POT, VEGETARIAN**

This recipe pays tribute to the wonderful cuisine of Louisiana and helps illustrate the diversity of bountiful Southern lands. Southern cooking has a bad reputation for being a heavier or unhealthy cuisine because traditionally long workdays and tough schedules once called for calorie-dense meals. This style of cooking draws inspiration from all across the world and deserves its place in the pantheon of American dining.

**2 tablespoons extra-virgin olive oil**

**½ large onion, chopped**

**1 pound collard greens, chopped**

**1 garlic clove, minced**

**½ teaspoon cayenne**

**3 cups low-sodium vegetable broth**

**2 tomatoes, diced**

1. Heat the extra-virgin olive oil in a large stockpot over medium heat. Sauté the onion until slightly softened and translucent, about 2 minutes.
2. Add the collards, garlic, and cayenne and cook for 2 to 3 minutes. Add the vegetable broth, cover, and bring the mixture to a simmer.
3. Simmer until the greens are tender, about 15 minutes. Add the tomatoes, adjust the seasonings as desired, and serve.
4. Store any leftovers in an airtight container in the refrigerator for 3 to 4 days.

**MAKE IT EASIER:** This dish also tastes great with canned tomatoes instead of fresh. If substituting, add one cup along with the vegetable broth.

**Per serving:** Calories: 127; Total fat: 8g; Carbohydrates: 13g; Fiber: 6g; Protein: 4g; Calcium: 290mg; Vitamin D: 0mcg; Vitamin $B_{12}$: 0mcg; Iron: 1mg; Zinc: <1mg

# Mashed Sweet Potatoes

*Serves 6 to 8 / Prep time: 10 minutes / Cook time: 20 minutes*

**GLUTEN-FREE, VEGETARIAN**

Personally, I love the peels in my mashed potatoes, but you may prefer to omit them. There's more fiber in the peel, so try cooking the potatoes with the skins first to get that extra nutrition in. And yes, there's butter in this recipe. I'm sorry, but it's not mashed potatoes without *some* butter. As long as you are pairing this side dish with foods that are low in saturated fat (lean meats and plants), then butter can be part of a balanced diet.

**2 medium sweet potatoes, cut into 1- to 2-inch cubes**

**4 medium carrots, cut into 1-inch cubes**

**6 garlic cloves, halved**

**¼ teaspoon kosher salt**

**2 tablespoons unsalted butter**

**⅓ cup unsweetened almond milk**

**Freshly ground black pepper**

1. Place the potatoes, carrots, garlic, and salt in a large stockpot and cover them with water by 1½ inches. Bring to a boil over high heat, reduce the heat to medium-high, and simmer for 10 to 15 minutes, until the vegetables become tender.
2. Drain the vegetables and return them to the pot. Add the butter and almond milk and mash until smooth with a potato masher. Season with pepper. Thin out with water or more milk to reach the desired consistency. Serve.
3. Store any leftovers in an airtight container in the refrigerator for up to 4 days.

**VARIATION:** Need more variety for your taste buds? Here are some of my favorite sweet potato mash-ups—be sure to try them all.

**Miso + ginger**

**Molasses + sesame seeds**

**Ginger + lime**

**Curry + coconut**

**Per serving:** Calories: 94; Total fat: 4g; Carbohydrates: 14g; Fiber: 3g; Protein: 1g; Calcium: 57mg; Vitamin D: <1mcg; Vitamin $B_{12}$: <1mcg; Iron: 1mg; Zinc: <1mg

# Charred Miso Cabbage

*Serves 4 / Prep time: 5 minutes / Cook time: 20 minutes*

**5-INGREDIENT, GLUTEN-FREE, HIGH-FIBER, VEGETARIAN**

This is one of my absolute favorite small plates to make for myself and to share. The combination of flavors and the added punch that comes from charring is a culinary journey you will want to take again and again. The meaty, crunchy nature of the cabbage adapts very well to grilling; you might never make this vegetable any other way.

**3 tablespoons avocado oil**

**1 head green cabbage, cut into 8 wedges**

**3 tablespoons yellow or white miso**

**2 tablespoons rice wine vinegar**

**1 lime, cut into 8 wedges**

1. Preheat the oven to 400°F. Line a baking sheet with parchment paper.
2. Heat the avocado oil in a large cast-iron pan or skillet over high heat. Arrange 2 or 3 cabbage wedges in the skillet and cook for about 3 minutes on each side until charred or lightly blackened. When they're seared on both sides, place the wedges on the baking sheet.
3. Repeat with the remaining wedges.
4. In a small bowl, mix the miso with the rice wine vinegar and brush it on the cabbage wedges evenly. Bake the wedges for 10 minutes.
5. When the wedges come out of the oven, squeeze the lime juice on them. Serve.
6. Store any leftovers in an airtight container in the refrigerator for 2 to 3 days.

**SUBSTITUTION TIP:** You've probably figured it out by now—that I'd tell you any vinegar will work just fine for this recipe. My first choice would be white wine, then cider, before distilled white vinegar. Use another plant-based oil in place of avocado if you prefer as well.

---

**Per serving:** Calories: 178; Total fat: 11g; Carbohydrates: 18g; Fiber: 6g; Protein: 5g; Calcium: 104mg; Vitamin D: 0mcg; Vitamin $B_{12}$: <1mcg; Iron: 2mg; Zinc: 1mg

# Avocado Slaw

*Serves 4 to 6 / Prep time: 15 minutes*

GLUTEN-FREE, HIGH-FIBER, NO-COOK, VEGETARIAN

Avocado is a nutrient-dense food that is full of heart-healthy fat, and it belongs on more than just toast. It's also incredibly creamy and makes an ideal substitute for mayonnaise and other common ingredients found in dressings. This is a very versatile recipe. It can be enjoyed on its own as a salad or side or added to the Jackfruit Tacos (page 103), the Game-Day Burger (page 80), or the Turkey Pastrami and Pimento Cheese Sandwich (page 79).

**1 avocado**

**⅓ cup water**

**3 tablespoons apple cider vinegar**

**1 tablespoon Dijon mustard**

**4 cups packed shredded cabbage (red, green, or mixed)**

**2 cups shredded carrot**

**Kosher salt**

**Freshly ground black pepper**

1. Place the avocado, water, vinegar, and mustard in a blender and puree until smooth. Add water if needed until you've reached a thin consistency, making the dressing easy to toss with the shredded vegetables.
2. In a large bowl, toss the cabbage and carrot with the dressing. Season to taste with salt and pepper and serve.
3. Store any leftovers in an airtight container in the refrigerator for up to 3 days.

**VARIATION:** Add other veggies to the slaw, like kale or jicama, to mix it up.

**Per serving:** Calories: 101; Total fat: 6g; Carbohydrates: 13g; Fiber: 6g; Protein: 2g; Calcium: 53mg; Vitamin D: 0mcg; Vitamin $B_{12}$: 0mcg; Iron: 1mg; Zinc: 1mg

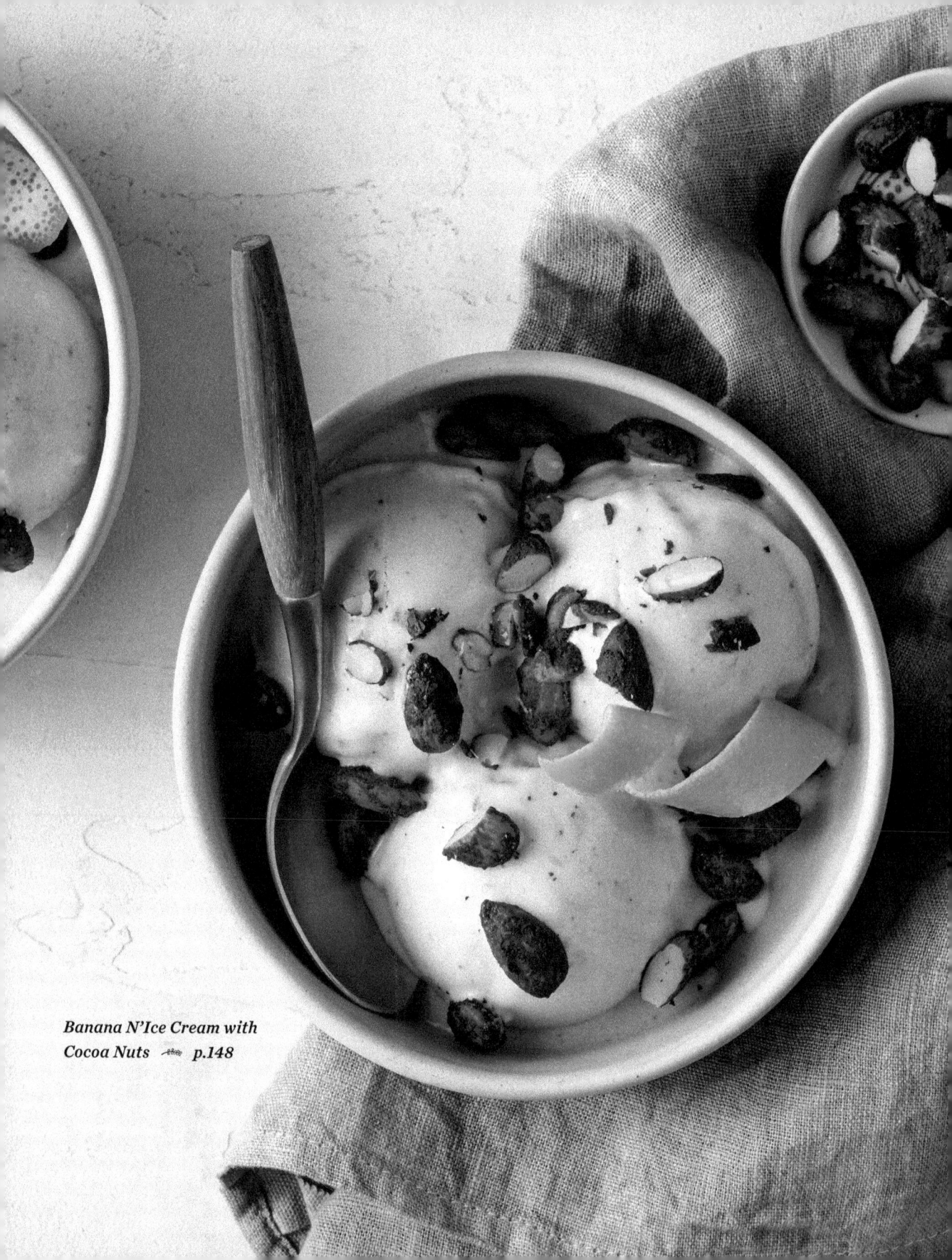

*Banana N'Ice Cream with Cocoa Nuts* p.148

CHAPTER EIGHT

# Dessert

Finally, the chapter you've been waiting for since the beginning of the book! You've probably heard that sugar and sweets are your enemies. But the chief philosophy of this book remains that everything can be enjoyed *in moderation*. This applies to sweets, too. There is no reason to cut your favorite things out of your diet entirely, nor is it necessary to deny yourself the things that bring you joy. What I mean to say is, you don't have to sacrifice dessert to live a healthy life.

In this chapter, I introduce recipes that will satisfy any sweet tooth without sugar overload or too many saturated fats. Dessert is the most important component of a meal for some people, a joyous treat deserving of celebration. This chapter has everything you need to enjoy dessert in its entirety while still maintaining a balanced diet.

Watermelon-Lime Granita ..... 147

Banana N'Ice Cream with Cocoa Nuts ..... 148

Blueberry Chocolate Clusters ..... 150

Superfood Brownie Bites ..... 151

Poached Pears ..... 152

Orange Praline with Yogurt ..... 153

Coconut Macaroons ..... 154

Chocolate Tahini Bombs ..... 155

# Watermelon-Lime Granita

*Serves 10 / Prep time: 15 minutes / Freeze time: 2½ hours*

**5-INGREDIENT, GLUTEN-FREE, NO-COOK, VEGETARIAN**

Cool and refreshing, this granita is perfect for the hot days of summer. While this recipe is quick and easy to make, it does require a bit of preplanning for it to taste best. The pureed fruit takes about 2½ hours to freeze and turn into a delicious slush, so make sure you plan ahead if serving this dessert.

**1 pound seedless watermelon flesh, cut into 1-inch chunks**

**2 tablespoons agave syrup**

**2 tablespoons freshly squeezed lime juice**

1. Line a baking sheet with parchment paper. Spread the watermelon chunks in a single layer on the sheet and freeze for at least 20 minutes.
2. Once the chunks are frozen, transfer them to a blender with the agave syrup and lime juice. Blend until liquefied and pour the mixture into a 9-by-13-inch shallow baking dish. Return to the freezer and freeze for 2 hours.
3. Every 30 minutes or so, take a fork and scrape the crystals into a slush consistency. Keep in the freezer for up to 1 month.

**VARIATION:** Surprise your palate and guests by adding a pinch of cayenne or chili powder to make the granita spicy. Substitute another type of citrus for the lime and different kinds of melon to create refreshing variations.

**Per serving:** Calories: 27; Total fat: <1g; Carbohydrates: 7g; Fiber: <1g; Protein: <1g; Calcium: 4mg; Vitamin D: 0mcg; Vitamin $B_{12}$: 0mcg; Iron: <1mg; Zinc: <1mg

# Banana N'Ice Cream with Cocoa Nuts

*Serves 4 to 6 / Prep time: 10 minutes / Cook time: 12 minutes*

**GLUTEN-FREE, HIGH-FIBER, VEGETARIAN**

It seems like everyone has frozen bananas on hand, and boy do they pile up quickly. If you are in danger of a frozen banana avalanche every time you open the freezer, this is the recipe for you. If your frozen bananas are whole, you will have to give them a rough chop before adding them to the food processor. If you don't have any frozen bananas, slice fresh bananas into small pieces, freeze them for 3 hours or overnight, then follow the recipe.

### FOR THE COCOA NUTS

**¼ cup freshly squeezed orange juice**

**1 tablespoon coconut oil**

**2 teaspoons cocoa powder**

**½ teaspoon kosher salt**

**¼ teaspoon ground cinnamon**

**¼ teaspoon ground cardamom**

**½ teaspoon orange zest**

**1 cup raw almonds**

### FOR THE BANANA N'ICE CREAM

**2 frozen, diced bananas**

### TO MAKE THE COCOA NUTS

1. Preheat the oven to 350°F. Line a baking sheet with parchment paper.
2. In a small saucepan, bring the orange juice to a boil over medium-high heat, reduce the heat to low, and simmer until the juice is reduced to about 2 tablespoons, 5 to 7 minutes. Add the coconut oil, stir until well combined, and remove from the heat. Whisk in the cocoa powder, salt, cinnamon, cardamom, and zest. Then add the almonds and stir to coat them. Spread the mixture onto the prepared baking sheet.
3. Bake the nuts for 10 to 12 minutes, stirring halfway through, until toasted. Allow to cool.
4. Store the nuts in an airtight container at room temperature for up to 2 weeks.

### TO MAKE THE BANANA N'ICE CREAM

5. Put the frozen bananas in a food processor and pulse. Scrape down the sides, then pulse once more. Continue to do this for several minutes until the texture resembles ice cream. Serve immediately with the cooled nuts.

**MAKE IT EASIER:** Skip the nuts and only make the banana n'ice cream; that way, you only need one ingredient for a delectable dessert!

**Per serving:** Calories: 333; Total fat: 24g; Carbohydrates: 23g; Fiber: 6g; Protein: 8g; Calcium: 122mg; Vitamin D: 0mcg; Vitamin $B_{12}$: 0mcg; Iron: 2mg; Zinc: <1mg

# Blueberry Chocolate Clusters

*Serves 10 / Prep time: 5 minutes / Cook time: 5 minutes*

**5-INGREDIENT, GLUTEN-FREE, VEGETARIAN**

We all grew up with Hershey's Kisses, and anyone who's ever been in a store around Valentine's Day has seen them in abundance. Making your own version is incredibly easy, and you don't have to wait for a holiday to enjoy them. Chocolate and blueberries are full of anti-oxidants and can help boost brain health.

**1½ cups dark chocolate chips**
**½ cups chopped, toasted pecans**
**2 cups blueberries**
**1 tablespoon coconut oil, melted**

1. Line a baking sheet with parchment paper.
2. Melt the chocolate in a microwave-safe bowl in 20- to 30-second intervals.
3. In a medium bowl, combine the melted chocolate with the coconut oil and pecans.
4. Spoon a small amount of chocolate mixture (about 1 teaspoon) on the prepared baking sheet.
5. Place a cluster of about 5 blueberries on top of the chocolate. You should get about 20 clusters in total.
6. Drizzle a small amount of chocolate over the berries.
7. Freeze until set, about 15 minutes.
8. Store in an airtight container in the refrigerator for up to 5 days or in the freezer for up to 1 month.

**VARIATION:** Any and all berries will do in these pretty clusters, and if you have any available, use a variety such as golden berry, raspberry, or mulberry. You could ditch the berries altogether and add other fresh fruit. Just be sure to cut the fruit into ¼-inch to ½-inch pieces.

**Per serving:** Calories: 230; Total fat: 17g; Carbohydrates: 18g; Fiber: 4g; Protein: 3g; Calcium: 26mg; Vitamin D: 0mcg; Vitamin $B_{12}$: <1mcg; Iron: 4mg; Zinc: 1mg

# Superfood Brownie Bites

*Makes 30 / Prep time: 15 minutes*

GLUTEN-FREE, NO-COOK, VEGETARIAN

Words like "superfood" get tossed around often and, in most cases, without justification. What exactly qualifies an ingredient as a superfood? In this case, it's the combination of nuts, seeds, cacao, and naturally sweet dates, all of which offer benefits to your body. Show up to any party with a platter of these brownie bites and watch them disappear.

**1 cup raw nuts (walnuts, pecans, or cashews)**
**½ cup hulled hemp seeds**
**⅓ cup raw pepitas**
**½ cup raw cacao powder**
**1 cup pitted dates**
**2 tablespoons coconut oil**
**1 teaspoon vanilla extract**

1. Line a baking sheet with parchment paper.
2. Place the nuts, hemp seeds, and pepitas in a food processor and pulse until the ingredients are a meal consistency. Add the cacao powder, dates, coconut oil, and vanilla extract and pulse until the mixture holds together if you pinch it with your fingers. The dough should ball up and appear glossy, and not be too sticky and wet. If it doesn't stick together enough to form a dough consistency, add water in drops until the correct consistency is reached. Be careful not to add too much liquid. If you do, add more cacao to balance the texture.
3. Scoop out the brownie bite mixture in 1-tablespoon amounts and roll the mixture into balls. Set the balls on the baking sheet and then chill them in the refrigerator for at least 10 minutes to hold their shape.
4. Transfer the balls to a container with a lid and store in the refrigerator until ready to eat. You could eat these immediately, but they are more likely to crumble.
5. Store brownies in an airtight container in the refrigerator for 5 to 7 days.

**MAKE IT EASIER:** Make a double or triple batch of brownies and freeze them. If stored in an airtight container in the freezer, these balls will keep for at least 1 month. Simply pop one out of the freezer when you want a nibble of something sweet.

**Per 1-bite serving:** Calories: 86; Total fat: 6g; Carbohydrates: 7g; Fiber: 2g; Protein: 3g; Calcium: 14mg; Vitamin D: 0mcg; Vitamin $B_{12}$: 0mcg; Iron: 1mg; Zinc: 1mg

# Poached Pears

*Serves 4 / Prep time: 10 minutes / Cook time: 20 minutes*

**GLUTEN-FREE, HIGH-FIBER, ONE-POT, VEGETARIAN**

Choosing fruit for dessert over sugar-filled pastries, cakes, and pies is a clear choice if you're looking to cut back on carbohydrates and calories, because whole fruit has more fiber and nutrients. Enjoy these spiced pears, which are poached to tasty perfection.

**2 cups white wine, preferably dry**

**1 cinnamon stick**

**1 (2-inch) piece of ginger, sliced**

**5 cardamom pods**

**Zest and juice of 2 oranges**

**4 Bosc pears, peeled, cored, and quartered**

1. Cut a piece of parchment paper into a circle slightly smaller in size than the saucepan you are using, and punch a small hole in its center.
2. In the medium saucepan, stir together the white wine, cinnamon, ginger, cardamom, and orange zest and juice on high heat. Bring to just before a boil, lower the heat so the liquid simmers, and add the pears.
3. Place the parchment paper over the pears. (This will keep just enough pressure for the pears to stay beneath the level of the poaching liquid and still allow steam to escape.)
4. Poach the pears for at least 20 minutes. The more time you have, the more flavor they will absorb.
5. Remove the pears from poaching liquid with a slotted spoon. Eat as is or return the poaching liquid (without the pears) to a simmer until the liquid reduces to a syrupy sauce, about 10 minutes. Strain the sauce and pour it over the poached pears.
6. Store the pears in an airtight container in the refrigerator for up to 4 days.

**INGREDIENT TIP:** My choice of pear for poaching would be a Bosc pear for both its flavor and ability to hold its shape during the poaching process, although the Anjou, Concorde, and French butter pears are also quite lovely. Avoid Comice and Bartlett pears if you can when making this recipe, as they don't hold up as well.

**Per serving:** Calories: 228; Total fat: <1g; Carbohydrates: 35g; Fiber: 6g; Protein: 1g; Calcium: 33mg; Vitamin D: 0mcg; Vitamin $B_{12}$: 0mcg; Iron: 1 mg; Zinc: <1mg

# Orange Praline with Yogurt

*Serves 6 / Prep time: 10 minutes / Cook time: 10 minutes*

**GLUTEN-FREE, ONE-POT, VEGETARIAN**

We have to thank the French immigrants who settled in Louisiana in the 19th century for introducing praline to the American South. Combine oranges, another staple of Southern desserts, and Greek yogurt as a substitute for cream, and voilà, you have a delicious dessert ready-made for those looking to cut back on carbohydrates.

**3 tablespoons sugar**
**4 teaspoons water**
**⅓ cup slivered almonds, toasted**
**½ teaspoon ground cinnamon**
**⅛ teaspoon ground cloves**
**1 tablespoon orange zest** (optional)
**Pinch kosher salt**
**3 cups plain Greek yogurt**

1. Preheat the oven to 375°F. Line a baking sheet with parchment paper.
2. In a small saucepan, stir together the sugar and water and cook over high heat until light golden-brown in color, 3 to 4 minutes. Do not stir, but instead gently swirl to help the sugar dissolve. Add the almonds and cook for 1 minute. The goal is to coat the almonds with the heated sugar (think caramel here) without burning. Pour the mixture onto the prepared baking sheet and set aside to cool for about 5 minutes.
3. Meanwhile, in a medium bowl, stir together the cinnamon, cloves, orange zest (if using), and salt.
4. Break the praline into smaller pieces and toss them in the spices.
5. Evenly divide the yogurt among six bowls and serve topped with the spiced praline. Store the praline in a sealed container at room temperature for up to 2 weeks.

**INGREDIENT TIP:** The praline can be sprinkled over anything creamy (frozen yogurt) or fruity (grilled peaches or fresh strawberries), so feel free to add it in moderation to your own creations.

**Per serving:** Calories: 163; Total fat: 8g; Carbohydrates: 12g; Fiber: 1g; Protein: 12g; Calcium: 154mg; Vitamin D: <1mcg; Vitamin $B_{12}$: <1mcg; Iron: <1mg; Zinc: 1mg

# Coconut Macaroons

*Makes 12 / Prep time: 10 minutes / Cook time: 20 minutes*

**VEGETARIAN**

Macaroons are an ancient treat traced all the way back to the Italian aristocracy of the 9th century. These cookies remain popular at dinner parties and celebrations today. The balanced flavors of the macaroon are timeless: delicate almond and coconut with a touch of sweetness. Whip up a batch of these treats when you're looking for a delicious dessert that doesn't have as much sugar as some of the more modern choices.

**1⅓ cups unsweetened shredded coconut**

**⅓ cup granulated sugar**

**2 tablespoons all-purpose flour**

**⅛ teaspoon kosher salt**

**2 large egg whites, at room temperature**

**½ teaspoon almond extract**

1. Preheat the oven to 325°F. Line a baking sheet with parchment paper.
2. In a small bowl, stir together the coconut, sugar, flour, and salt until well combined. Create a well in the center and add the egg whites and almond extract. Mix the two together, then slowly mix the egg white mixture into the coconut mixture.
3. Spoon the batter onto the baking sheet in 1-tablespoon amounts, making about 12 cookies in total. If they aren't rounded, use your hands to gently roll each into a ball.
4. Bake the cookies for 18 to 20 minutes, until golden brown. Allow to cool and enjoy.
5. Store the cookies at room temperature in an airtight container for up to 1 week.

**VARIATION:** Coffee or vanilla extract can be used in place of the almond extract. You can also fold in different nuts if you want more of a crunch to the cookie.

**Per 1-macaroon serving:** Calories: 98; Total fat: 7g; Carbohydrates: 9g; Fiber: 2g; Protein: 2g; Calcium: 7mg; Vitamin D: <1mcg; Vitamin $B_{12}$: <1mcg; Iron: 1mg; Zinc: <1mg

# Chocolate Tahini Bombs

*Makes 15 each / Prep time: 20 minutes / Cook time: 8 minutes*

**5-INGREDIENT, GLUTEN-FREE, VEGETARIAN**

Sesame is the unsung hero of the dessert world and a healthier way to enjoy something sweet. Tahini, the ground product of toasted sesame seeds, contains more protein than milk and most nuts. This fragrant paste is a rich source of B vitamins, which boost energy and brain function; vitamin E, which helps fight heart disease and stroke; and minerals like magnesium, iron, and calcium. It's amazing to find all of this nutritional power in a simple dessert.

**15 whole dates, pits removed (date intact, not split in half completely)**

**2½ tablespoons tahini, divided**

**½ cup canned coconut milk**

**4 ounces dark chocolate, chopped**

**1 tablespoon toasted sesame seeds**

1. Line a baking sheet with parchment paper.
2. Fill each date with a small amount of the tahini, roughly ¼ teaspoon, and place them on the prepared baking sheet. Put the filled dates in the freezer for 10 to 15 minutes.
3. Meanwhile, heat the coconut milk in a small saucepan over medium-low until simmering.
4. Place the chocolate in a medium heatproof bowl, and when the milk is simmering, pour it into the bowl and let stand for 3 minutes to soften the chocolate.
5. Stir the mixture until it is smooth and the chocolate is completely melted.
6. Remove the dates from the freezer and dip one date at a time into the chocolate. Coat evenly using a fork and place them back on the baking sheet. Sprinkle the dates with the sesame seeds and repeat until all dates are coated in chocolate.
7. Allow to cool completely for the chocolate to harden, or eat immediately.

**INGREDIENT TIP:** If the chocolate is not melting, do not put it in the microwave! Place the bowl in a saucepan filled with a few inches of gently simmering water over low heat and stir the chocolate until it melts.

**Per 1-tahini-bomb serving:** Calories: 97; Total fat: 6g; Carbohydrates: 10g; Fiber: 2g; Protein: 1g; Calcium: 20mg; Vitamin D: 0mcg; Vitamin $B_{12}$: <1mcg; Iron: 1mg; Zinc: <1mg

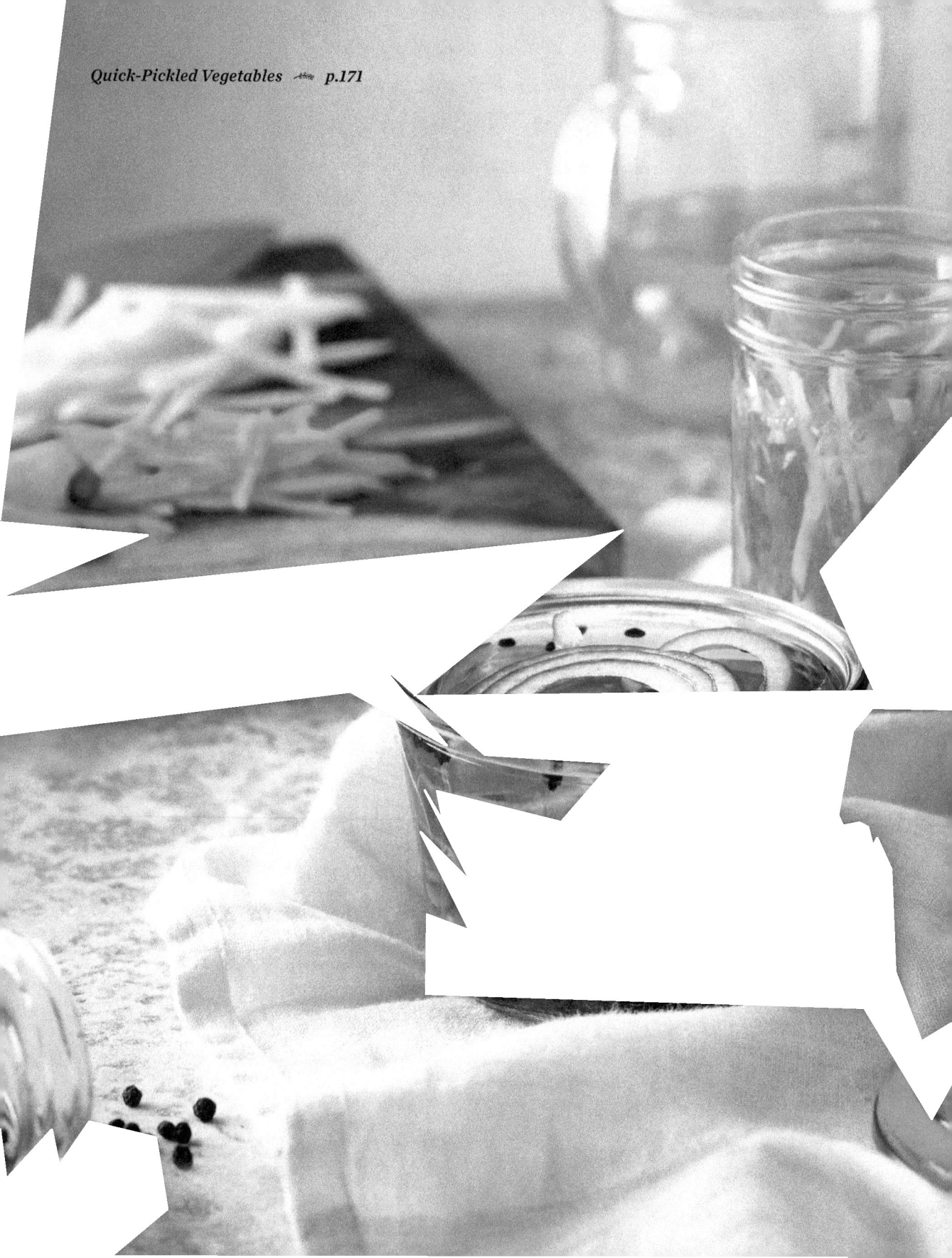

*Quick-Pickled Vegetables* p.171

CHAPTER NINE

# Seasonings, Sauces, and Dressings

This chapter contains all the seasonings, sauces, and dressings that bring out the best in the recipes I've covered in this book. A tasty dish has many components, and it is the relationship between those components—the way each ingredient works with another—that creates perfection on the plate. Over the years, I've enjoyed experimenting and playing around with how tastes work together—for example, what spice blend produces a chorus of unique flavors, how much oil to blend or salt to add to a salad dressing, or what sauce complements a beautiful cut of meat or grain bowl. It is my hope that this chapter not only gives you the tools you need to make my seasonings, sauces, and dressings, but also inspires you to play around with your own ideas. Cooking is a journey after all, and this chapter is here to guide you on the next step.

Lemon Vinaigrette Dressing ..... 159

Chile-Lime Dressing ..... 160

Poppy Seed Dressing ..... 161

Tahini Dressing ..... 162

Caesar Dressing, Two Ways ..... 163

Cherry Barbecue Sauce ..... 165

Basic Marinara ..... 166

Tomato, Caper, and Golden Raisin Sauce ..... 167

Peanut Sauce ..... 168

Harissa ..... 169

Romesco Sauce ..... 170

Quick-Pickled Vegetables ..... 171

# Lemon Vinaigrette Dressing

*Makes 1 cup / Prep time: 5 to 10 minutes*

**GLUTEN-FREE, NO-COOK, ONE BOWL, VEGETARIAN**

Here is a basic lemon vinaigrette recipe that is versatile and super easy to make. In fact, it's so easy, you'll never want to buy it premade again! The fresh lemon juice is key, so be sure to avoid the premade, shelf-stable juice in the grocery aisle. It cannot compete with fresh in this case. Use the vinaigrette as a marinade, drizzle it over roasted vegetables, toss it with a cooked grain, or use it in place of other dressings.

**¼ cup freshly squeezed lemon juice**

**2 garlic cloves, minced**

**1 teaspoon Dijon mustard**

**½ teaspoon maple syrup** (optional)

**¼ cup extra-virgin olive oil**

**½ cup grapeseed oil**

**Kosher salt**

**Freshly ground black pepper**

1. In a small bowl, whisk together the lemon juice, garlic, mustard, and maple syrup (if using). Slowly whisk in the extra-virgin olive oil, followed by the grapeseed oil, until the dressing is completely emulsified. Season with salt and pepper to taste.
2. Store the dressing in an airtight container for up to 1 week in the refrigerator or in the freezer for up to 3 months.

**INGREDIENT TIP:** Grapeseed oil has a neutral flavor, which is why I often combine it with a good-tasting extra-virgin olive oil in my salad dressings. Sometimes extra-virgin olive oil alone can taste grassy, so adding another neutral oil can balance it out. That said, you can replace the grapeseed oil with additional extra-virgin olive oil.

**Per 2-tablespoon serving:** Calories: 184; Total fat: 20g; Carbohydrates: 1g; Fiber: <1g; Protein: <1g; Calcium: 2mg; Vitamin D: 0mcg; Vitamin $B_{12}$: 0mcg; Iron: <1mg; Zinc: <1mg

# Chile-Lime Dressing

*Makes 1 cup / Prep time: 5 minutes*

GLUTEN-FREE, NO-COOK, ONE BOWL

This dressing is so dynamic and flavorful you don't really need much else in your salad. It brings life into the simplest of greens. However, the dressing doesn't need to be limited to salad alone. You can try it on fish, chicken, roasted vegetables, and rice with stellar results.

**5 ounces grapeseed or safflower oil**

**Zest and juice of 4 limes**

**4 garlic cloves, minced**

**4-inch piece fresh ginger, minced**

**2½ tablespoons chile paste**

**2 teaspoons fish sauce** (optional)

**¼ teaspoon kosher salt**

1. Combine the grapeseed oil, lime zest and juice, garlic, ginger, chile paste, fish sauce (if using), and salt in a jar or container with a tight-fitting lid. Close the lid and shake the mixture vigorously to combine.
2. Store the dressing in an airtight container for up to 1 week in the refrigerator or in the freezer for up to 3 months.

**MAKE IT EASIER:** Use the back of a spoon to peel the ginger, and make sure you roll the lime before zesting and juicing. Rolling breaks open the cells that release the juice.

**Per 2-tablespoon serving:** Calories: 179; Total fat: 18g; Carbohydrates: 6g; Fiber: <1g; Protein: <1g; Calcium: 6mg; Vitamin D: 0mcg; Vitamin $B_{12}$: 0mcg; Iron: <1mg; Zinc: <1mg

# Poppy Seed Dressing

*Makes 1 cup / Prep time: 5 minutes*

GLUTEN-FREE, NO-COOK, ONE POT, VEGETARIAN

There's a sweetness to this dressing that is addictive but also comforting; it reminds me of something my grandmother used to make in her small kitchen in northern Minnesota. But even if you're not from the Midwest, this dressing can conjure up a vision of cozy family dinners. These meals highlight the beauty of cooking and eating together.

**½ cup plain Greek yogurt**
**¼ cup white wine vinegar**
**3 tablespoons grapeseed oil**
**2 tablespoons Dijon mustard**
**1 tablespoon honey**
**1 small shallot, minced**
**1½ tablespoons poppy seeds**

1. In a blender, puree the yogurt, vinegar, grapeseed oil, mustard, honey, and shallot. Transfer to a container or jar with a lid and stir in the poppy seeds. If you don't have a blender, mix by hand in a medium bowl using a whisk *or* add to a jar with a fitted lid and shake vigorously.
2. Store the dressing in an airtight container for up to 1 week in the refrigerator or in the freezer for up to 3 months.

**VARIATION:** Use a neutral oil such as canola in place of the grapeseed oil for a different flavor profile.

**Per 2-tablespoon serving:** Calories: 83; Total fat: 7g; Carbohydrates: 4g; Fiber: 1g; Protein: 2g; Calcium: 44mg; Vitamin D: 0mcg; Vitamin $B_{12}$: <1mcg; Iron: <1mg; Zinc: <1mg

# Tahini Dressing

*Makes 1 cup / Prep time: 5 minutes*

**GLUTEN-FREE, NO-COOK, ONE BOWL, VEGETARIAN**

Tahini dressing is one of those special ingredients that can be used for almost anything: Dinner? Sure, pour it across anything from steak to chicken or rice to just about any vegetable. Dessert? Well, if you've tried the Chocolate Tahini Bombs on page 155, you'll understand its sweeter side as well. I also like to use tahini dressing for breakfast as a topping for fresh greens and a soft-boiled egg on the side.

**⅔ cup filtered water**

**⅓ cup tahini**

**¼ cup freshly squeezed lemon juice (about 2 lemons)**

**1 tablespoon extra-virgin olive oil**

**2 teaspoons maple syrup**

**Kosher salt**

**Freshly ground black pepper**

1. In a small bowl, whisk together the water, tahini, lemon juice, extra-virgin olive oil, and maple syrup. Season to taste with salt and pepper. Adjust the consistency by adding more water or extra-virgin olive oil.
2. Store the dressing in an airtight container for up to 1 week in the refrigerator or in the freezer for up to 3 months.

**VARIATION:** Try honey, agave, or even molasses in place of maple syrup. These sweeteners all balance the dressing and add a unique taste.

**Per 2-tablespoon serving:** Calories: 81; Total fat: 7g; Carbohydrates: 4g; Fiber: 1g; Protein: 2g; Calcium: 45mg; Vitamin D: 0mcg; Vitamin $B_{12}$: 0mcg; Iron: 1mg; Zinc: <1mg

# Caesar Dressing, Two Ways

*Makes ~1½ cups of each dressing / Prep time: 5 minutes*

GLUTEN-FREE (CHECK WORCESTERSHIRE), NO-COOK, ONE-POT

Caesar salad has made its way into the pantheon of American staples. Very few restaurants, whether a steakhouse, Italian taverna, or grab-and-go joint, omit this dish from the menu. I've developed a couple of different ways to enjoy it here—a classic, lighter version and a vegan version—both of which allow you to enjoy its rich, umami goodness while keeping things focused on health.

## For the Classic Light Version

**1 cup plain Greek yogurt**

**¼ cup freshly squeezed lemon juice (about 2 lemons)**

**4 anchovy fillets, coarsely chopped**

**2 tablespoons Dijon mustard**

**2 tablespoons extra-virgin olive oil**

**3 garlic cloves, peeled**

**1 teaspoon Worcestershire sauce**

**Pinch freshly ground black pepper**

1. Place the yogurt, lemon juice, anchovies, mustard, extra-virgin olive oil, garlic, Worcestershire, and pepper in a blender and puree until smooth. Adjust the seasonings as desired.
2. Store in an airtight container for 5 to 7 days, or in the freezer for up to 3 months.

continued

## For the Vegan Version

**½ cup raw sunflower seeds, soaked in water for 2 hours or overnight**

**¼ cup extra-virgin olive oil**

**3 tablespoons freshly squeezed lemon juice**

**2 garlic cloves, minced**

**1 tablespoon nutritional yeast**

**1 tablespoon tahini**

**1 teaspoon Dijon mustard**

**1 teaspoon maple syrup**

**½ teaspoon tamari**

1. Drain the sunflower seeds and place them in a blender with the extra-virgin olive oil, lemon juice, garlic, nutritional yeast, tahini, mustard, maple syrup, and tamari. Blend until smooth. If the dressing is too thick, slowly stream in cold water as the machine is running and blend until smooth. Adjust the seasonings as desired.
2. Store in an airtight container in the refrigerator for 5 to 7 days or in the freezer for up to 3 months.

**MAKE IT EASIER:** Both versions of this dressing will keep for at least 1 week if stored in the fridge or for 1 month in the freezer, so double it up to have extra for those times you don't want to cook.

**Classic Light Version per 2-tablespoon serving:** Calories: 44; Total fat: 3g; Carbohydrates: 2g; Fiber: <1g; Protein: 2g; Calcium: 26mg; Vitamin D: 0mcg; Vitamin $B_{12}$: <1mcg; Iron: <1mg; Zinc: <1mg

**Vegan Version per 2-tablespoon serving:** Calories: 87; Total fat: 8g; Carbohydrates: 3g; Fiber: 1g; Protein: 2g; Calcium: 12mg; Vitamin D: 0mcg; Vitamin $B_{12}$: 1mcg; Iron: 1mg; Zinc: <1mg

# Cherry Barbecue Sauce

*Makes 2 cups / Prep time: 5 minutes*

GLUTEN-FREE, NO-COOK, ONE POT, VEGETARIAN

Is there anything more American than barbecue? It's essential for lazy summer nights with neighbors or family gatherings on the Fourth of July. If you grew up with a grill as a staple cooking method as I did, just the smell of a good barbecue sauce would evoke powerful memories of time spent with people you love. This sweet, tangy cherry barbecue sauce honors these memories while helping create new ones as well.

**10 ounces pitted fresh cherries**
**1 small onion, quartered**
**2 tablespoons Dijon mustard**
**2 tablespoons red wine vinegar**
**1 tablespoon ground fennel seeds**
**3 chipotle peppers in adobo sauce, plus 1 tablespoon sauce**
**Pinch freshly ground black pepper**

1. In a blender, combine the cherries, onion, mustard, vinegar, fennel, chipotle peppers, adobo sauce, and black pepper. Puree until combined and adjust the seasonings as desired.
2. Store in an airtight container in the refrigerator for up to 1 week or in the freezer for up to 3 months.

**MAKE IT EASIER:** Frozen cherries are an excellent substitute for the fresh ones in this recipe, but you must thaw the fruit beforehand. The best part is that they come pitted, saving you the effort.

**Per ¼-cup serving:** Calories: 39; Total fat: 1g; Carbohydrates: 8g; Fiber: 2g; Protein: 1g; Calcium: 18mg; Vitamin D: 0mcg; Vitamin $B_{12}$: 0mcg; Iron: <1mg; Zinc: <1mg

# Basic Marinara

*Makes 8 cups / Prep time: 5 minutes / Cook time: 25 minutes*

GLUTEN-FREE, ONE POT, VEGETARIAN

What is left to say about marinara that hasn't already been said? There's a reason why classic pasta and pizza recipes still call for this ode to fresh tomatoes and basil. The beauty of great dishes often lies in their simplicity and balance. In this recipe, I add just enough garlic, oregano, and black pepper to hit the right spot every time.

**¼ cup extra-virgin olive oil**
**1 small onion, minced**
**4 garlic cloves, thinly sliced**
**2 basil sprigs**
**1 teaspoon dried oregano**
**2 (28-ounce) cans diced or crushed tomatoes**
**Kosher salt**
**Freshly ground pepper**

1. Heat the extra-virgin olive oil in a medium heavy stockpot over medium heat. Cook the onion, stirring occasionally, until very soft, 3 to 5 minutes.
2. Add the garlic and cook, stirring occasionally, until very soft, about 5 minutes. Add the basil and oregano and stir to combine.
3. Add the tomatoes and bring to a simmer. Reduce the heat to low and simmer, stirring occasionally, until the sauce is thick, about 15 minutes.
4. Season with salt and pepper.
5. Store in an airtight container in the refrigerator for up to 1 week or in the freezer for up to 3 months.

**MAKE IT EASIER:** Having extra tomato sauce available is lovely, which is why this recipe makes 8 cups. Store the extra in an airtight container in the freezer if you don't plan to eat all of it within 5 days. Otherwise, you could cut the recipe in half.

**Per ½-cup serving:** Calories: 59; Total fat: 3g; Carbohydrates: 6g; Fiber: 2g; Protein: 1g; Calcium: 4mg; Vitamin D: 0mcg; Vitamin $B_{12}$: 0mcg; Iron: <1mg; Zinc: <1mg

# Tomato, Caper, and Golden Raisin Sauce

*Makes ~4 cups / Prep time: 5 minutes / Cook time: 25 minutes*

**GLUTEN-FREE, ONE-POT, VEGETARIAN**

Although this Mediterranean-based sauce is used in the Cauliflower Steaks recipe (page 104), it also pairs beautifully with meats like beef, lamb, or chicken and even fish like swordfish and halibut. One could also use it in place of marinara sauce when making pasta for a little more sweetness and an enticing, distinct dish.

**2 tablespoons extra-virgin olive oil**

**6 garlic cloves, minced**

**1 (28-ounce) can crushed tomatoes**

**¼ cup golden raisins**

**2 tablespoons capers**

**1 teaspoon dried oregano**

**Pinch kosher salt**

**Pinch freshly ground black pepper**

**3 fresh basil leaves**

1. Heat the extra-virgin olive oil in a large saucepan over medium heat. Sauté the garlic until softened, about 3 minutes. Add the tomatoes, raisins, capers, oregano, salt, and pepper and bring the sauce to a simmer. Add the basil leaves, including the stem, and allow them to wilt, then submerge the leaves in the sauce.
2. Simmer the sauce until thickened, about 15 minutes.
3. Store in an airtight container in the refrigerator for up to 1 week or in the freezer for up to 3 months.

**VARIATION:** Make the sauce even more exciting with the addition of salty anchovies, olives, or dried herbs such as marjoram, tarragon, parsley, or thyme.

**Per ½-cup serving:** Calories: 82; Total fat: 4g; Carbohydrates: 12g; Fiber: 2g; Protein: 2g; Calcium: 46mg; Vitamin D: 0mcg; Vitamin $B_{12}$: 0mcg; Iron: 2mg; Zinc: <1mg

# Peanut Sauce

*Makes 1 to 1¼ cups / Prep time: 5 to 10 minutes*

**HIGH-FIBER, NO-COOK, ONE BOWL, VEGETARIAN**

Peanut butter, and peanuts, in general, have gotten a lot of love over the years. Peanut sauce is used in pan-Asian dishes, especially those developed by Thai and Laotian immigrants and other members of the Southeast Asian diaspora. These exotic dishes prepare peanuts in a way you maybe hadn't seen before. This peanut sauce is a nod to this tradition and works well on everything, such as noodles, chicken, salad, and rice.

**½ cup unsalted, unsweetened creamy peanut butter**

**2 tablespoons soy or tamari sauce**

**1 tablespoon honey**

**2 garlic cloves, minced**

**1 teaspoon diced chile**

**Juice of 1 lime**

1. In a medium bowl, whisk together the peanut butter, soy sauce, honey, garlic, chile, and lime juice until thoroughly combined. Add water to thin out the consistency. Taste and adjust the seasonings as desired.
2. Store in an airtight container in the refrigerator for up to 1 week or in the freezer for up to 3 months.

**VARIATION:** Add 1 teaspoon of fish sauce or grated ginger if you'd like to try something with more of an umami, or rich and savory, flavor.

**Per ¼-cup serving:** Calories: 426; Total fat: 34g; Carbohydrates: 20g; Fiber: 6g; Protein: 17g; Calcium: 47mg; Vitamin D: 0mcg; Vitamin $B_{12}$: 0mcg; Iron: 2mg; Zinc: <1mg

# Harissa

*Makes 2½ cups / Prep time: 15 to 20 minutes / Cook time: 10 minutes*

**GLUTEN-FREE, VEGETARIAN**

Harissa is a North African hot chile pepper paste, the main ingredients of which are roasted red peppers, spices, and herbs. This paste has a kick—it fills your mouth immediately with a bright, fiery flavor. I've toned this recipe down a bit by swapping out the spicier peppers for red bell peppers, although you can still use those hotter ingredients. This does not diminish the quality of the condiment one bit, so it will brighten up your plate.

**1 tablespoon coriander seeds**
**1 tablespoon caraway seeds**
**4 red bell peppers**
**4 large garlic cloves**
**½ cup extra-virgin olive oil**
**2 teaspoons red pepper flakes**
**Kosher salt**
**Freshly ground black pepper**

1. In a small skillet over medium-high heat, toast the coriander and caraway for about 30 seconds. Transfer the mixture to a mortar and pestle or spice grinder and grind into powder.
2. Char the bell peppers over a gas flame, in a cast-iron pan, or under the broiler until blackened, about 3 minutes on each side. If using an open flame, rotate and turn each pepper so that the entire pepper chars. Then place the peppers in a medium bowl, cover the bowl with plastic wrap, and let stand for 5 to 10 minutes. When the peppers are cool enough to handle, peel, seed, and put them in a food processor. Add the toasted spices, garlic, extra-virgin olive oil, and red pepper flakes and pulse to form a uniform paste. Season the harissa with salt and pepper to taste.
3. Store in an airtight container in the refrigerator for 5 to 7 days or in the freezer for up to 3 months.

**MAKE IT EASIER:** Skip the toasting process altogether and use ground spices instead of whole.

**Per ¼-cup serving:** Calories: 189; Total fat: 19g; Carbohydrates: 7g; Fiber: 3g; Protein: 1g; Calcium: 23mg; Vitamin D: 0mcg; Vitamin $B_{12}$: 0mcg; Iron: 1mg; Zinc: <1mg

# Romesco Sauce

*Makes ~2 cups / Prep time: 5 to 10 minutes*

HIGH-FIBER, NO-COOK, ONE BOWL, VEGETARIAN

Romesco is a tomato-based sauce that comes originally from Catalonia. It might not be quite as well-known as marinara, but it's just as delicious and, in many ways, a bolder culinary ingredient. This recipe will become a go-to favorite with its combination of sherry vinegar, cayenne pepper, paprika, and almond blended with the natural brightness of fresh tomato.

**3 roasted red bell peppers**
**2 slices toasted whole-wheat bread, cubed**
**1 medium tomato**
**5 garlic cloves**
**½ cup toasted almonds**
**2 tablespoons sherry vinegar**
**1 tablespoon smoked paprika**
**¼ teaspoon kosher salt**
**¼ teaspoon cayenne pepper**
**¼ cup extra-virgin olive oil**

1. In a food processor, combine the bell peppers, bread, tomato, garlic, almonds, sherry vinegar, paprika, salt, and cayenne. Puree and then, while the machine is running, slowly stream in the extra-virgin olive oil. Stop the machine, taste, and adjust the seasonings as desired.
2. Store in an airtight container in the refrigerator for up to 1 week or in the freezer for up to 3 months.

**VARIATION:** Swap out the sherry vinegar for others such as cider, white, champagne, or even red wine vinegar.

**Per ½-cup serving:** Calories: 310; Total fat: 24g; Carbohydrates: 19g; Fiber: 5g; Protein: 8g; Calcium: 101mg; Vitamin D: 0mcg; Vitamin $B_{12}$: 0mcg; Iron: 2mg; Zinc: 1mg

# Quick-Pickled Vegetables

Pickles are a great item to keep on hand for many reasons. They are incredibly versatile and can be put on the burger and many other recipes mentioned in this book. You can also use them as a complement to any rice or grain bowl. I like to eat them by themselves after letting the vegetables sit in the brine, because they taste even better the longer they soak. This simple recipe can be stored up to 1 month in the refrigerator, so there's no rush to eat them right away.

## Pickled Red Onions

*Makes 1½ cups / Prep time: 3 minutes*

5-INGREDIENT, GLUTEN-FREE, NO-COOK, ONE BOWL, VEGETARIAN

**1 red onion, thinly sliced**

**1 cup cider vinegar**

**1 tablespoon whole black peppercorns** (optional)

1. In a small bowl, combine the red onion with the cider vinegar and black peppercorns. Allow the onions to marinate for at least 15 minutes and up to 1 hour at room temperature.
2. Serve immediately or store in the refrigerator in an airtight container for up to 1 week.

continued

## Pickled Carrot and Radish

*Makes 2 cups / Prep time: 10 minutes*

GLUTEN-FREE, NO-COOK, ONE BOWL, VEGETARIAN

**1 cup warm water**
**2 tablespoons granulated sugar**
**1 cup carrots, julienne cut or sliced with a peeler**
**1 cup radish, preferably daikon, julienne cut or sliced with a peeler**
**1 cup rice wine vinegar**
**½ teaspoon kosher salt**

1. In a small bowl, whisk together the water and sugar. Add the carrots, radish, vinegar, and salt. Set aside and allow to marinate for at least 15 minutes and up to one hour at room temperature.
2. Serve immediately or store in the refrigerator in an airtight container for up to 1 week.

**VARIATION:** Adjust the flavor by adding whole spices to either quick pickle. Try fennel seed, dill, mustard seed, or black peppercorns.

**Pickled onions per ½-cup serving:** Calories: 20; Total fat: <1g; Carbohydrates: 5g; Fiber: 1g; Protein: 1g; Calcium: 12mg; Vitamin D: 0mcg; Vitamin $B_{12}$: 0mcg; Iron: <1mg; Zinc: <1mg

**Pickled carrots per ½-cup serving:** Calories: 45; Total fat: <1g; Carbohydrates: 11g; Fiber: 2g; Protein: 1g; Calcium: 22mg; Vitamin D: 0mcg; Vitamin $B_{12}$: 0mcg; Iron: <1mg; Zinc: <1mg

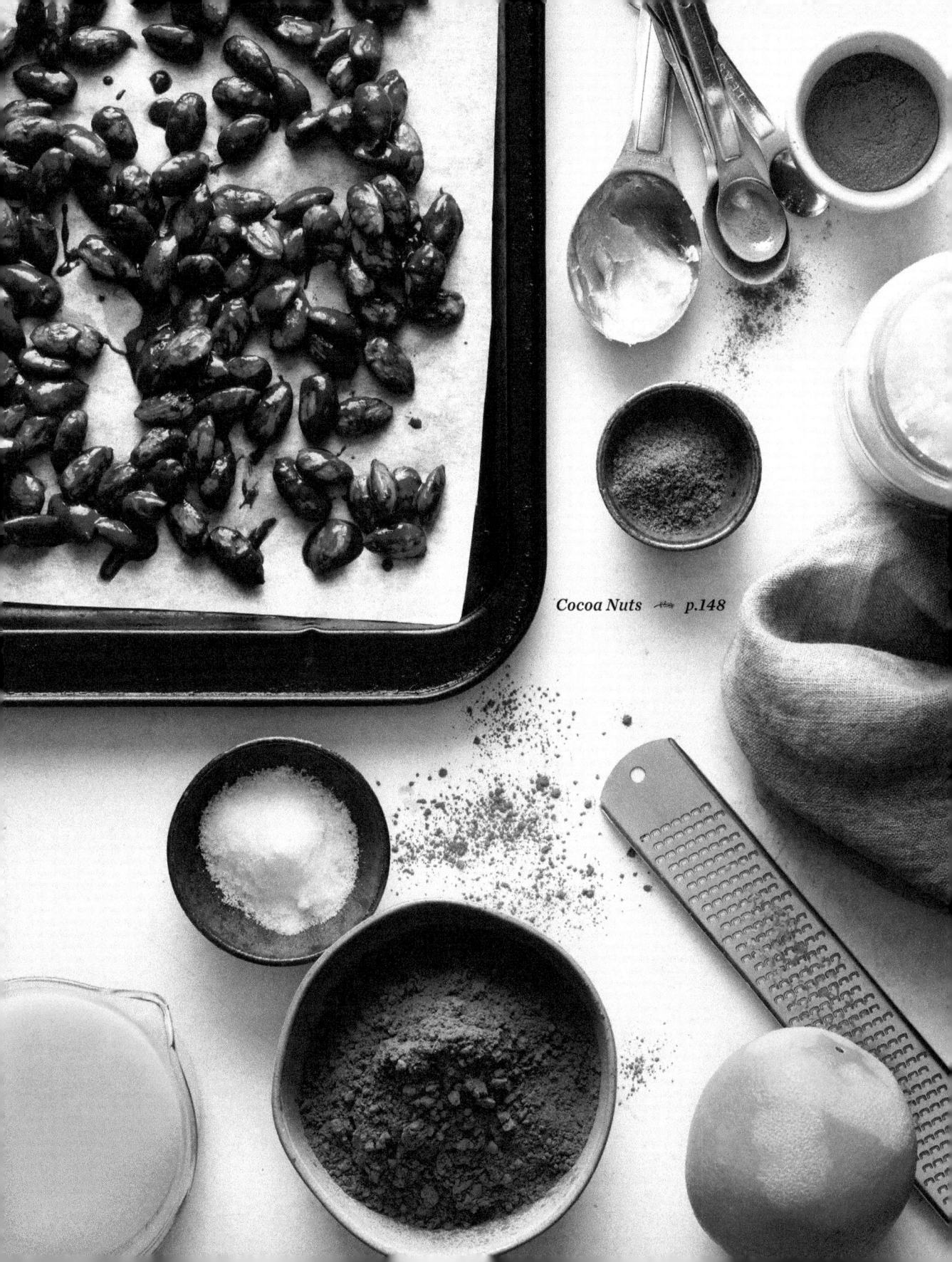

*Cocoa Nuts* p.148

# Measurement Conversions

| Volume Equivalents | US STANDARD | US STANDARD (OUNCES) | METRIC (APPROXIMATE) |
|---|---|---|---|
| Liquid | 2 tablespoons | 1 fl. oz. | 30 mL |
| | ¼ cup | 2 fl. oz. | 60 mL |
| | ½ cup | 4 fl. oz. | 120 mL |
| | 1 cup | 8 fl. oz. | 240 mL |
| | 1½ cups | 12 fl. oz. | 355 mL |
| | 2 cups or 1 pint | 16 fl. oz. | 475 mL |
| | 4 cups or 1 quart | 32 fl. oz. | 1 L |
| | 1 gallon | 128 fl. oz. | 4 L |
| Dry | ⅛ teaspoon | — | 0.5 mL |
| | ¼ teaspoon | — | 1 mL |
| | ½ teaspoon | — | 2 mL |
| | ¾ teaspoon | — | 4 mL |
| | 1 teaspoon | — | 5 mL |
| | 1 tablespoon | — | 15 mL |
| | ¼ cup | — | 59 mL |
| | ⅓ cup | — | 79 mL |
| | ½ cup | — | 118 mL |
| | ⅔ cup | — | 156 mL |
| | ¾ cup | — | 177 mL |
| | 1 cup | — | 235 mL |
| | 2 cups or 1 pint | — | 475 mL |
| | 3 cups | — | 700 mL |
| | 4 cups or 1 quart | — | 1 L |
| | ½ gallon | — | 2 L |
| | 1 gallon | — | 4 L |

## Oven Temperatures

| FAHRENHEIT | CELSIUS (APPROXIMATE) |
|---|---|
| 250°F | 120°C |
| 300°F | 150°C |
| 325°F | 165°C |
| 350°F | 180°C |
| 375°F | 190°C |
| 400°F | 200°C |
| 425°F | 220°C |
| 450°F | 230°C |

## Weight Equivalents

| US STANDARD | METRIC (APPROXIMATE) |
|---|---|
| ½ ounce | 15 g |
| 1 ounce | 30 g |
| 2 ounces | 60 g |
| 4 ounces | 115 g |
| 8 ounces | 225 g |
| 12 ounces | 340 g |
| 16 ounces or 1 pound | 455 g |

# Resources

It can be a challenge to know where to go for factual information. If you don't see a specific resource listed below, there are many—be sure to look for professionals who specialize in diabetes and nutrition, such as MDs, endocrinologists, certified diabetes care and education specialists, and registered dietitians.

## Books

*Body Kindness* by Rebecca Scritchfield, RDN

*Dr. Bernstein's Diabetes Solution: The Complete Guide to Achieving Normal Blood Sugars* by Richard K. Bernstein, MD

*Intuitive Eating* by Evelyn Tribole, MS, RDN, and Elyse Resch, MS, RDN, CEDRD-S, FAND

## Websites

CDC.gov/diabetes/ndep/people-risk-diabetes/index.html

DiabetesEducator.org

Diabetes.org

## Apps for Your Phone

Diabetes Tracker (Apple)

Glucose Buddy (Apple and Android)

Health2Sync (Apple and Android)

MyFitnessPal (Apple and Android)

MyNetDiary's Diabetes Tracker (Android)

mySugr (Apple and Android)

Noom (Apple and Android)

# References


Academy of Nutrition and Dietetics. "Carbohydrates–Part of a Healthful Diabetes Diet." EatRight.org. Published January 28, 2019. EatRight.org/health/diseases-and-conditions/diabetes/carbohydrates-part-of-a-healthful-diabetes-diet.

American Association of Diabetes Educators 2014. *The Art & Science of Diabetes Self-Management Education Desk Reference*, 3rd ed. Chicago, IL: AADE, 2014.

American Diabetes Association. "Standards of Medical Care in Diabetes—2021." *The Journal of Clinical and Applied Research and Education.* Volume 44, Supplement (January 2021.) S1–S2. doi.org/10.2337/dc20-Sint.

Association of Diabetes Care & Education Specialists. "AADE7 Self-Care Behaviors." Accessed February 3, 2020. DiabetesEducator.org/living-with-diabetes/aade7-self-care-behaviors.

Astbury, Nerys M., Moira A. Taylor, and Ian A. Macdonald. "Breakfast Consumption Affects Appetite, Energy Intake, and the Metabolic and Endocrine Responses to Foods Consumed Later in the Day in Male Habitual Breakfast Eaters." *The Journal of Nutrition* 141, no. 7 (July 2011): 1381–1389. doi.org/10.3945/jn.110.128645.

Atkinson, Fiona S., Kaye Foster-Powell, and Jennie C. Brand-Miller. "International Tables of Glycemic Index and Glycemic Load Values: 2008." *Diabetes Care* 31, no. 12 (December 2008): 2281–2283. doi.org/10.2337/dc08-1239.

Banihani, Saleem Ali. "Radish (*Raphanus sativus*) and Diabetes." *Nutrients* 9, no. 9 (June 2017): 1014. doi.org/10.3390/nu9091014.

Berg, Christina, Georgios Lappas, Alicja Wolk, Elisabeth Strandhagen, Kjell Torén, Annika Rosengren, Dag Thelle, and Lauren Lissner. "Eating Patterns and Portion Size Associated with Obesity in a Swedish Population." *Appetite* 52, no. 1 (February 2009): 21–26. doi.org/10.1016/j.appet.2008.07.008.

Centers for Disease Control and Prevention. "National Diabetes Statistics Report, 2017." CDC.gov, Updated July 17, 2017. Accessed January 31, 2020. CDC.gov/diabetes/data/statistics/statistics-report.html.

Diabetes Prevention Program Research Group. "Long-term Effects of Lifestyle Intervention or Metformin on Diabetes Development and Microvascular Complications over 15-Year Follow-up: The Diabetes Prevention Program Outcomes Study." *The Lancet: Diabetes & Endocrinology* 3, no. 11 (November 2015): 866–875. doi.org/10.1016/S2213-8587(15)00291-0.

Evert, Alison B., et al. "Nutrition Therapy for Adults with Diabetes or Prediabetes: A Consensus Report." *Diabetes Care* 42, no. 5 (May 2019): 731–754. doi.org/10.2337/dci19-0014.

Fraser, Claire E., Donald J. D'Amico, et al. "Diabetic Retinopathy: Prevention and Treatment." UpToDate.com. Last updated October 29, 2019. UpToDate.com/contents/diabetic-retinopathy-prevention-and-treatment.

Giovannini, Marcello, Carlo Agostoni, and Raanan Shamir. "Symposium Overview: Do We All Eat Breakfast and Is It Important?" *Critical Reviews in Food Science and Nutrition* 50, no. 2 (January 2010): 97–99. doi.org/10.1080/10408390903467373.

Glycemic Index Foundation. "About Glycemic Index." Accessed February 3, 2020. GISymbol.com/about-glycemic-index.

Golan, A., I. Wolman, J. Sagi, et al. "Persistence of Polyhydramnios During Pregnancy–Its Significance and Correlation with Maternal and Fetal Complications." *Gynecologic and Obstetric Investigation* 37, no. 1 (1994): 18–20. doi.org/10.1159/000292513.

Goyal, Raksha and Sandeep Julka. "Impact of Breakfast Skipping on the Health Status of the Population." *Indian Journal of Endocrinology and Metabolism* 18, no. 5 (September–October 2014): 683–687. NCBI.NLM.NIH.gov/pmc/articles/PMC4171892.

Hostalek, Ulrike. "Global Epidemiology of Prediabetes—Present and Future Perspectives." *Clinical Diabetes and Endocrinology* 5, no. 5 (May 9, 2019). NCBI.NLM.NIH.gov/pmc/articles/PMC6507173.

Iowa State University. "Brain Activity Helps Explain Diabetics' Negative Feelings, Risk for Depression." ScienceDaily.com. Published May 2018. ScienceDaily.com/releases/2018/05/180507111821.htm.

Kutsuma, Ayano, Kei Nakajima, and Kaname Suwa. "Potential Association between Breakfast Skipping and Concomitant Late-Night-Dinner Eating with Metabolic Syndrome and Proteinuria in the Japanese Population." *Scientifica* 2014, no. 253581 (2014). doi.org/10.1155/2014/253581.

Leidy, Heather J. "The Benefits of Breakfast Consumption to Combat Obesity and Diabetes in Young People." *American Journal of Lifestyle Medicine* 7, no. 2 (November 29, 2012): 99–103. doi.org/10.1177/1559827612468687.

McCrory, Megan A. and Wayne W. Campbell. "Effects of Eating Frequency, Snacking, and Breakfast Skipping on Energy Regulation: Symposium Overview." *The Journal of Nutrition* 141, no. 1 (January 2011): 144–147. doi.org/10.3945/jn.109.114918.

Mintel Press Team. "A Snacking Nation: 94% of Americans Snack Daily." Mintel.com. Published July 9, 2015. Mintel.com/press-centre/food-and-drink/a-snacking-nation-94-of-americans-snack-daily.

"Natural Medicines." Natural Medicines in the Clinical Management of Diabetes website. Accessed January 31, 2020. NaturalDatabase.TherapeuticResearch.com/ce/CECourse.aspx?cs=naturalstandard&s=ND&pm=5&pc18-110.

Pike, Alyssa. "Snacking on the Rise: 2019 Food & Health Survey Results." FoodInsight.org. Published May 31, 2019. FoodInsight.org/snacking-on-the-rise-2019-food-health-survey-results.

Slavin, Joanne and Justin Carlson. "Carbohydrates." *Advances in Nutrition* 5, no. 6 (November 2014): 760–761. doi.org/10.3945/an.114.006163.

St-Onge, Marie-Pierre, et al. "Meal Timing and Frequency: Implications for Cardiovascular Disease Prevention: A Scientific Statement from the American Heart Association." *Circulation* 135 (2017): e96–e121. doi.org/10.1161/CIR.0000000000000476.

Wolf, Tovah, Vera Tsenkova, Carol D. Ryff, Richard J. Davidson, and Auriel A. Willette. "Neural, Hormonal, and Cognitive Correlates of Metabolic Dysfunction and Emotional Reactivity." *Psychosomatic Medicine* 80, no. 5: (June 2018): 452–459. doi.org/10.1097/PSY0000000000000582.

Wyatt, Holly R., Gary K. Grunwald, Cecilia L. Mosca, Mary L. Klem, Rena R. Wing, and James O. Hill. "Long-term Weight Loss and Breakfast in Subjects in the National Weight Control Registry." *Obesity Research* 10, no. 2 (February 2002): 78–82. doi.org/10.1038/oby.2002.13.

# Index


## A

Almonds
- Banana N'Ice Cream with Cocoa Nuts, 148–149
- Cherry, Chocolate, and Almond Shake, 34
- Orange Praline with Yogurt, 153
- Roasted Asparagus with Romesco Sauce, 133–134
- Romesco Sauce, 170
- Spinach Salad with Strawberries and Toasted Almonds, 57

Apples
- Apple-Bulgur Salad, 64
- Apple Millet Porridge, 40

Apricots, Chicken Salad with, 76

Asparagus
- Asparagus Salad with Chile-Lime Dressing, 58
- Red Lentil Sloppy Joes with Roasted Asparagus, 78
- Roasted Asparagus with Romesco Sauce, 133–134

Avocados
- Avocado Slaw, 142
- Avocado-Tofu Scramble with Roasted Potatoes, 50–51
- Citrus Avocado Salad, 55

## B

Bacon, Ribboned Squash with, 110

Bananas
- Banana N'Ice Cream with Cocoa Nuts, 148–149
- Breakfast Banana Barley, 41
- Tahini, Maple, and Banana Overnight Oats, 38

Barley, Breakfast Banana, 41

Basic Marinara, 166

Beans, 19
- Grilled Romaine with White Beans, 66
- Lemony White Bean Puree, 130
- Smoked Turkey Chili, 91

Beef
- Game-Day Burger with Jicama Chips, 80–81
- Lebanese-Inspired Beef Kebabs with Pickled Onions, 112–113
- Miso Skirt Steak, 118

Beet Grain Bowl, Sweet, 65

Bell peppers
- Roasted Asparagus with Romesco Sauce, 133–134
- Romesco Sauce, 170
- Shakshuka, 47

Berries, 19
- Blueberry-Chia Smoothie, 33
- Blueberry Chocolate Clusters, 150
- Harvest Blackberry Quinoa Bowl, 42
- Spinach Salad with Strawberries and Toasted Almonds, 57
- Strawberry-Ricotta Toast, 45

Bibimbap, Simple, 101

Blackberry Quinoa Bowl, Harvest, 42

Blueberries
- Blueberry-Chia Smoothie, 33
- Blueberry Chocolate Clusters, 150

Bowls
- Harvest Blackberry Quinoa Bowl, 42
- Sweet Beet Grain Bowl, 65
- Tuna Poke with Riced Broccoli, 105–106

Breakfast Banana Barley, 41

Breakfast, importance of, 21

Broccoli
Charred Sesame Broccoli, 135
Sautéed Lemon Broccoli and Kale, 132
Tuna Poke with Riced Broccoli, 105–106
Brownie Bites, Superfood, 151
Brussels Sprouts, Shaved, and Kale with Poppy Seed Dressing, 62
Buckwheat Crêpes, Easy, 46
Buckwheat Noodles, Peanut Tofu over, 100
Bulgur-Apple Salad, 64
Burger, Game-Day, with Jicama Chips, 80–81

## C

Cabbage
Avocado Slaw, 142
Charred Miso Cabbage, 141
Caesar Dressing, Two Ways, 163–164
Cajun-Style Collards, 139
Capers
Cauliflower Steaks with Tomato, Caper, and Golden Raisin Sauce, 104
Tomato, Caper, and Golden Raisin Sauce, 167
Carbohydrates, 6–7, 15–17, 28
Carrots
Carrot Cake Oatmeal, 44
Miso, Tempeh, and Carrot Wraps, 75
Pickled Carrot and Radish, 172
Roasted Carrot and Chickpea Dip, 127
Roasted Carrot and Quinoa with Goat Cheese, 68
Cauliflower
Cauliflower Rice, 138
Cauliflower Steaks with Tomato, Caper, and Golden Raisin Sauce, 104
Cauli-Lettuce Wraps, 74
Chicken Sausage and Cauliflower Pizza, 120
Pomegranate "Tabbouleh" with Cauliflower, 61
Simple Bibimbap, 101
Charred Miso Cabbage, 141
Charred Sesame Broccoli, 135
Cheese
Roasted Carrot and Quinoa with Goat Cheese, 68
Strawberry-Ricotta Toast, 45
Tomato-Basil Soup with Grilled Cheese Croutons, 84–85
Turkey Pastrami and Pimento Cheese Sandwich, 79
Vegetable Mac 'n' Cheese, 102
Cherries
Cherry Barbecue Chicken Cutlets, 116–117
Cherry Barbecue Sauce, 165
Cherry, Chocolate, and Almond Shake, 34
Chia-Blueberry Smoothie, 33
Chicken
Cherry Barbecue Chicken Cutlets, 116–117
Chicken Khao Sen with Rice Noodles, 111
Chicken Salad with Apricots, 76
Chicken Sausage and Cauliflower Pizza, 120
Golden Chicken Soup, 90
Herbed Buttermilk Chicken, 119
Quick Moroccan-Inspired Chicken Stew, 92
Chickpeas
Chickpea Fattoush Salad, 67
Chickpea Spinach Soup, 88–89
Roasted Carrot and Chickpea Dip, 127
Turkey Bolognese with Chickpea Pasta, 121
Chile-Lime Dressing, 160
Chocolate
Banana N'Ice Cream with Cocoa Nuts, 148–149
Blueberry Chocolate Clusters, 150
Cherry, Chocolate, and Almond Shake, 34
Chocolate Tahini Bombs, 155
Superfood Brownie Bites, 151
Cholesterol, 17, 20
Citrus Avocado Salad, 55
Coconut Macaroons, 154

Collards, Cajun-Style, 139
Crêpes, Easy Buckwheat, 46
Cucumbers
  Cucumber Roll-Ups, 125
  Quinoa and Cucumber Salad, 63
  Smashed Cucumber Salad, 136
Curried Yogurt, Eggplant and Lentils with, 98–99

# D

Dairy products, 19
Desserts
  Banana N'Ice Cream with Cocoa Nuts, 148–149
  Blueberry Chocolate Clusters, 150
  Chocolate Tahini Bombs, 155
  Coconut Macaroons, 154
  Orange Praline with Yogurt, 153
  Poached Pears, 152
  Superfood Brownie Bites, 151
  Watermelon-Lime Granita, 147
Diabetes, 4, 5
Diabetes Prevention Program (DPP), 6
Diet
  foods to embrace, 19–20
  foods to moderate, 20
  mealtimes, 21
  modifications to, 6–7
  portion sizes, 21–22
  and prediabetes, 15–17
Dips and spreads
  Lemony White Bean Puree, 130
  Roasted Carrot and Chickpea Dip, 127
Doctors, questions to ask, 12
Dressings
  Caesar Dressing, Two Ways, 163–164
  Chile-Lime Dressing, 160
  Lemon Vinaigrette Dressing, 159
  Poppy Seed Dressing, 161
  Tahini Dressing, 162

# E

Easy Buckwheat Crêpes, 46
Eggplants
  Eggplant and Lentils with Curried Yogurt, 98–99
  Eggplant Breakfast Sandwich, 48
  Eggplant Pizzas, 126
Eggs
  Egg Drop Soup, 83
  Eggplant Breakfast Sandwich, 48
  Perfect Egg Scramble with Simple Salad, 49
  Shakshuka, 47
Equipment, 25–26
Exercise, 7–8

# F

Fats, 20
Fish and seafood
  Salmon en Papillote, 114–115
  Smoked Salmon on Toast, 77
  Tuna Poke with Riced Broccoli, 105–106
  Walnut-Crusted Halibut with Pear Salad, 107–108
5-ingredient
  Blueberry-Chia Smoothie, 33
  Blueberry Chocolate Clusters, 150
  Breakfast Banana Barley, 41
  Cauliflower Rice, 138
  Cauliflower Steaks with Tomato, Caper, and Golden Raisin Sauce, 104
  Charred Miso Cabbage, 141
  Charred Sesame Broccoli, 135
  Cherry Barbecue Chicken Cutlets, 116–117
  Cherry, Chocolate, and Almond Shake, 34
  Chicken Sausage and Cauliflower Pizza, 120
  Chocolate Tahini Bombs, 155
  Cucumber Roll-Ups, 125
  Easy Buckwheat Crêpes, 46
  Garlic Roasted Radishes, 137
  Harvest Blackberry Quinoa Bowl, 42

5-ingredient (*continued*)
High-Protein Oatmeal, 43
Pickled Red Onions, 171
Roasted Asparagus with Romesco Sauce, 133–134
Shaved Brussels Sprouts and Kale with Poppy Seed Dressing, 62
Spinach Salad with Strawberries and Toasted Almonds, 57
Strawberry-Ricotta Toast, 45
Watermelon-Lime Granita, 147
Freezer staples, 23

## G

Game-Day Burger with Jicama Chips, 80–81
Garlic Roasted Radishes, 137
Gestational diabetes (GDM), 5
Gingered Red Lentils with Millet, 97
Gluten-free
Apple Millet Porridge, 40
Asparagus Salad with Chile-Lime Dressing, 58
Avocado Slaw, 142
Avocado-Tofu Scramble with Roasted Potatoes, 50–51
Banana N'Ice Cream with Cocoa Nuts, 148–149
Basic Marinara, 166
Blueberry-Chia Smoothie, 33
Blueberry Chocolate Clusters, 150
Caesar Dressing, Two Ways, 163–164
Cajun-Style Collards, 139
Carrot Cake Oatmeal, 44
Cauliflower Rice, 138
Cauliflower Steaks with Tomato, Caper, and Golden Raisin Sauce, 104
Charred Miso Cabbage, 141
Cherry Barbecue Chicken Cutlets, 116–117
Cherry Barbecue Sauce, 165
Cherry, Chocolate, and Almond Shake, 34
Chicken Khao Sen with Rice Noodles, 111
Chicken Salad with Apricots, 76
Chicken Sausage and Cauliflower Pizza, 120
Chickpea Spinach Soup, 88–89
Chile-Lime Dressing, 160
Chocolate Tahini Bombs, 155
Citrus Avocado Salad, 55
Cucumber Roll-Ups, 125
Easy Buckwheat Crêpes, 46
Eggplant and Lentils with Curried Yogurt, 98–99
Eggplant Breakfast Sandwich, 48
Eggplant Pizzas, 126
Garlic Roasted Radishes, 137
Gingered Red Lentils with Millet, 97
Golden Chicken Soup, 90
Green Bean and Radish Potato Salad, 131
Grilled Romaine with White Beans, 66
Harissa, 169
Harvest Blackberry Quinoa Bowl, 42
Herbed Buttermilk Chicken, 119
Herbed Tomato Salad, 56
High-Protein Oatmeal, 43
Italian-Style Turkey Meatballs and Zoodles, 109
Jackfruit Tacos, 103
Kale Caesar Salad, 59–60
Kale Chip Nachos, 128–129
Lebanese-Inspired Beef Kebabs with Pickled Onions, 112–113
Lemon Vinaigrette Dressing, 159
Lemony White Bean Puree, 130
Mashed Sweet Potatoes, 140
Minted Sweet Pea Soup, 82
Miso, Tempeh, and Carrot Wraps, 75
Orange Praline with Yogurt, 153
Overnight Oats, 38–39
Peanut Tofu over Buckwheat Noodles, 100
Perfect Egg Scramble with Simple Salad, 49
Pickled Carrot and Radish, 172
Pickled Red Onions, 171

Poached Pears, 152
Pomegranate "Tabbouleh" with Cauliflower, 61
Poppy Seed Dressing, 161
Quick Moroccan-Inspired Chicken Stew, 92
Quinoa and Cucumber Salad, 63
Ribboned Squash with Bacon, 110
Roasted Carrot and Chickpea Dip, 127
Roasted Carrot and Quinoa with Goat Cheese, 68
Salmon en Papillote, 114–115
Sautéed Lemon Broccoli and Kale, 132
Seedy Muesli, 37
Shaved Brussels Sprouts and Kale with Poppy Seed Dressing, 62
Smashed Cucumber Salad, 136
Smoked Turkey Chili, 91
Spinach Salad with Strawberries and Toasted Almonds, 57
Superfood Brownie Bites, 151
Tahini Dressing, 162
Tahini, Maple, and Banana Overnight Oats, 38
Tomato-Basil Soup with Grilled Cheese Croutons, 84–85
Tomato, Caper, and Golden Raisin Sauce, 167
Tropical Mango Overnight Oats, 39
Turkey Bolognese with Chickpea Pasta, 121
Watermelon-Lime Granita, 147
West African–Inspired Peanut Soup, 86–87
Glycemic index (GI), 16
Goat Cheese, Roasted Carrot and Quinoa with, 68
Golden Chicken Soup, 90
Golden raisins
Cauliflower Steaks with Tomato, Caper, and Golden Raisin Sauce, 104
Tomato, Caper, and Golden Raisin Sauce, 167
Granita, Watermelon-Lime, 147
Granola, Stovetop, 35–36
Grapefruits
Citrus Avocado Salad, 55
Green Bean and Radish Potato Salad, 131
Greens, 19
Grilled Cheese Croutons, Tomato-Basil Soup with, 84–85
Grilled Romaine with White Beans, 66
Grocery shopping, 27

# H

Halibut, Walnut-Crusted, with Pear Salad, 107–108
Harissa, 169
Harvest Blackberry Quinoa Bowl, 42
Health-care providers, 12
Herbal supplements, 10–11
Herbed Buttermilk Chicken, 119
Herbed Tomato Salad, 56
High-fiber
Apple-Bulgur Salad, 64
Apple Millet Porridge, 40
Asparagus Salad with Chile-Lime Dressing, 58
Avocado Slaw, 142
Banana N'Ice Cream with Cocoa Nuts, 148–149
Blueberry-Chia Smoothie, 33
Breakfast Banana Barley, 41
Cajun-Style Collards, 139
Carrot Cake Oatmeal, 44
Cauliflower Steaks with Tomato, Caper, and Golden Raisin Sauce, 104
Cauli-Lettuce Wraps, 74
Charred Miso Cabbage, 141
Cherry, Chocolate, and Almond Shake, 34
Chicken Khao Sen with Rice Noodles, 111
Chickpea Fattoush Salad, 67
Chickpea Spinach Soup, 88–89
Citrus Avocado Salad, 55
Eggplant and Lentils with Curried Yogurt, 98–99

High-fiber (*continued*)
Eggplant Breakfast Sandwich, 48
Eggplant Pizzas, 126
Game-Day Burger with Jicama Chips, 80–81
Gingered Red Lentils with Millet, 97
Grilled Romaine with White Beans, 66
Harvest Blackberry Quinoa Bowl, 42
High-Protein Oatmeal, 43
Italian-Style Turkey Meatballs and Zoodles, 109
Jackfruit Tacos, 103
Kale Caesar Salad, 59–60
Kale Chip Nachos, 128–129
Lemony White Bean Puree, 130
Minted Sweet Pea Soup, 82
Miso, Tempeh, and Carrot Wraps, 75
Peanut Sauce, 168
Peanut Tofu over Buckwheat Noodles, 100
Poached Pears, 152
Pomegranate "Tabbouleh" with Cauliflower, 61
Quinoa and Cucumber Salad, 63
Red Lentil Sloppy Joes with Roasted Asparagus, 78
Ribboned Squash with Bacon, 110
Roasted Asparagus with Romesco Sauce, 133–134
Roasted Carrot and Quinoa with Goat Cheese, 68
Roasted Tomato Tartine, 73
Romesco Sauce, 170
Salmon en Papillote, 114–115
Sautéed Lemon Broccoli and Kale, 132
Seedy Muesli, 37
Shakshuka, 47
Shaved Brussels Sprouts and Kale with Poppy Seed Dressing, 62
Simple Bibimbap, 101
Smoked Turkey Chili, 91
Spinach Salad with Strawberries and Toasted Almonds, 57
Strawberry-Ricotta Toast, 45
Sweet Beet Grain Bowl, 65
Tomato-Basil Soup with Grilled Cheese Croutons, 84–85
Tuna Poke with Riced Broccoli, 105–106
Turkey Bolognese with Chickpea Pasta, 121
Vegetable Mac 'n' Cheese, 102
Walnut-Crusted Halibut with Pear Salad, 107–108
West African–Inspired Peanut Soup, 86–87
High-Protein Oatmeal, 43

## I

Ingredient staples, 23–25
Insulin resistance, 2, 5
Italian-Style Turkey Meatballs and Zoodles, 109

## J

Jackfruit Tacos, 103
Jicama Chips, Game-Day Burger with, 80–81

## K

Kale
Kale Caesar Salad, 59–60
Kale Chip Nachos, 128–129
Sautéed Lemon Broccoli and Kale, 132
Shaved Brussels Sprouts and Kale with Poppy Seed Dressing, 62
Kebabs, Lebanese-Inspired Beef, with Pickled Onions, 112–113

## L

Lebanese-Inspired Beef Kebabs with Pickled Onions, 112–113
Lemons
Lemon Vinaigrette Dressing, 159
Lemony White Bean Puree, 130
Sautéed Lemon Broccoli and Kale, 132

Lentils
Eggplant and Lentils with Curried Yogurt, 98–99
Gingered Red Lentils with Millet, 97
Red Lentil Sloppy Joes with Roasted Asparagus, 78
Lettuce
Cauli-Lettuce Wraps, 74
Grilled Romaine with White Beans, 66
Limes
Asparagus Salad with Chile-Lime Dressing, 58
Chile-Lime Dressing, 160
Watermelon-Lime Granita, 147

# M

Macaroons, Coconut, 154
Mac 'n' Cheese, Vegetable, 102
Mango Overnight Oats, Tropical, 39
Maple, Tahini, and Banana Overnight Oats, 38
Mashed Sweet Potatoes, 140
Meatballs, Italian-Style Turkey, and Zoodles, 109
Medications, 7
Metabolic syndrome, 21
Milks, plant-based, 20
Millet
Apple Millet Porridge, 40
Gingered Red Lentils with Millet, 97
Minted Sweet Pea Soup, 82
Miso
Charred Miso Cabbage, 141
Miso Skirt Steak, 118
Miso, Tempeh, and Carrot Wraps, 75
Muesli, Seedy, 37

# N

Nachos, Kale Chip, 128–129
No-cook
Asparagus Salad with Chile-Lime Dressing, 58
Avocado Slaw, 142
Blueberry-Chia Smoothie, 33
Caesar Dressing, Two Ways, 163–164
Cherry Barbecue Sauce, 165
Cherry, Chocolate, and Almond Shake, 34
Chicken Salad with Apricots, 76
Chile-Lime Dressing, 160
Citrus Avocado Salad, 55
Cucumber Roll-Ups, 125
Herbed Tomato Salad, 56
Lemon Vinaigrette Dressing, 159
Lemony White Bean Puree, 130
Overnight Oats, 38–39
Peanut Sauce, 168
Pickled Carrot and Radish, 172
Pickled Red Onions, 171
Poppy Seed Dressing, 161
Romesco Sauce, 170
Seedy Muesli, 37
Shaved Brussels Sprouts and Kale with Poppy Seed Dressing, 62
Smashed Cucumber Salad, 136
Smoked Salmon on Toast, 77
Spinach Salad with Strawberries and Toasted Almonds, 57
Strawberry-Ricotta Toast, 45
Superfood Brownie Bites, 151
Tahini Dressing, 162
Tahini, Maple, and Banana Overnight Oats, 38
Tropical Mango Overnight Oats, 39
Turkey Pastrami and Pimento Cheese Sandwich, 79
Watermelon-Lime Granita, 147
Noodles. *See also* Pasta
Chicken Khao Sen with Rice Noodles, 111
Peanut Tofu over Buckwheat Noodles, 100
Nutritional information, 28

## O

Oats
- Carrot Cake Oatmeal, 44
- High-Protein Oatmeal, 43
- Overnight Oats, 38–39
- Tahini, Maple, and Banana Overnight Oats, 38
- Tropical Mango Overnight Oats, 39

Omega-3 fatty acids, 19
One pot/pan/bowl
- Apple Millet Porridge, 40
- Basic Marinara, 166
- Blueberry-Chia Smoothie, 33
- Breakfast Banana Barley, 41
- Caesar Dressing, Two Ways, 163–164
- Cajun-Style Collards, 139
- Carrot Cake Oatmeal, 44
- Cauli-Lettuce Wraps, 74
- Cherry Barbecue Sauce, 165
- Cherry, Chocolate, and Almond Shake, 34
- Chicken Salad with Apricots, 76
- Chicken Sausage and Cauliflower Pizza, 120
- Chile-Lime Dressing, 160
- Citrus Avocado Salad, 55
- Cucumber Roll-Ups, 125
- Easy Buckwheat Crêpes, 46
- Golden Chicken Soup, 90
- Green Bean and Radish Potato Salad, 131
- Harvest Blackberry Quinoa Bowl, 42
- Herbed Buttermilk Chicken, 119
- Herbed Tomato Salad, 56
- High-Protein Oatmeal, 43
- Lemon Vinaigrette Dressing, 159
- Orange Praline with Yogurt, 153
- Overnight Oats, 38–39
- Peanut Sauce, 168
- Peanut Tofu over Buckwheat Noodles, 100
- Pickled Carrot and Radish, 172
- Pickled Red Onions, 171
- Poached Pears, 152
- Poppy Seed Dressing, 161
- Quick Moroccan-Inspired Chicken Stew, 92
- Romesco Sauce, 170
- Seedy Muesli, 37
- Shaved Brussels Sprouts and Kale with Poppy Seed Dressing, 62
- Smoked Turkey Chili, 91
- Spinach Salad with Strawberries and Toasted Almonds, 57
- Stovetop Granola, 35–36
- Strawberry-Ricotta Toast, 45
- Sweet Beet Grain Bowl, 65
- Tahini Dressing, 162
- Tahini, Maple, and Banana Overnight Oats, 38
- Tomato, Caper, and Golden Raisin Sauce, 167
- Tropical Mango Overnight Oats, 39
- Tuna Poke with Riced Broccoli, 105–106
- Turkey Pastrami and Pimento Cheese Sandwich, 79
- West African–Inspired Peanut Soup, 86–87

Onions
- Lebanese-Inspired Beef Kebabs with Pickled Onions, 112–113
- Pickled Red Onions, 171

Oranges
- Citrus Avocado Salad, 55
- Orange Praline with Yogurt, 153

Overnight Oats, 38–39

## P

Pantry staples, 23–25
Pasta
- Turkey Bolognese with Chickpea Pasta, 121
- Vegetable Mac 'n' Cheese, 102

Peanut butter
Peanut Sauce, 168
Peanut Tofu over Buckwheat Noodles, 100
West African-Inspired Peanut Soup, 86–87
Pears
Poached Pears, 152
Walnut-Crusted Halibut with Pear Salad, 107–108
Pea Soup, Minted Sweet, 82
Perfect Egg Scramble with Simple Salad, 49
Pickled Carrot and Radish, 172
Pickled Red Onions, 171
Pimento Cheese and Turkey Pastrami Sandwich, 79
Pizzas
Chicken Sausage and Cauliflower Pizza, 120
Eggplant Pizzas, 126
Poached Pears, 152
Pomegranate "Tabbouleh" with Cauliflower, 61
Poppy Seed Dressing, 161
Porridge, Apple Millet, 40
Portion sizes, 21–22
Potatoes
Avocado-Tofu Scramble with Roasted Potatoes, 50–51
Green Bean and Radish Potato Salad, 131
Prediabetes
about, 1–2
causes of, 2–4
diet and, 15–17
foods to embrace, 19–20
foods to moderate, 20
health effects of, 4
treatments for, 6–8

# Q

Quick Moroccan-Inspired Chicken Stew, 92
Quick-Pickled Vegetables, 171–172
Quinoa
Harvest Blackberry Quinoa Bowl, 42
Quinoa and Cucumber Salad, 63
Roasted Carrot and Quinoa with Goat Cheese, 68

# R

Radishes
Garlic Roasted Radishes, 137
Green Bean and Radish Potato Salad, 131
Pickled Carrot and Radish, 172
Recipes, about, 27–29
Red Lentil Sloppy Joes with Roasted Asparagus, 78
Refined foods, 20
Refrigerator staples, 23
Retinopathy, 4
Ribboned Squash with Bacon, 110
Rice Noodles, Chicken Khao Sen, 111
Ricotta-Strawberry Toast, 45
Risk factors, 2–4
Roasted Asparagus with Romesco Sauce, 133–134
Roasted Carrot and Chickpea Dip, 127
Roasted Carrot and Quinoa with Goat Cheese, 68
Roasted Tomato Tartine, 73
Romesco Sauce, 170

# S

Salads. *See also* Bowls; Dressings
Apple-Bulgur Salad, 64
Asparagus Salad with Chile-Lime Dressing, 58
Avocado Slaw, 142
Chicken Salad with Apricots, 76
Chickpea Fattoush Salad, 67
Citrus Avocado Salad, 55
Green Bean and Radish Potato Salad, 131
Grilled Romaine with White Beans, 66

Salads (*continued*)
Herbed Tomato Salad, 56
Kale Caesar Salad, 59–60
Perfect Egg Scramble with Simple Salad, 49
Pomegranate "Tabbouleh" with Cauliflower, 61
Quinoa and Cucumber Salad, 63
Roasted Carrot and Quinoa with Goat Cheese, 68
Shaved Brussels Sprouts and Kale with Poppy Seed Dressing, 62
Smashed Cucumber Salad, 136
Spinach Salad with Strawberries and Toasted Almonds, 57
Walnut-Crusted Halibut with Pear Salad, 107–108
Salmon
Salmon en Papillote, 114–115
Smoked Salmon on Toast, 77
Sandwiches and wraps
Cauli-Lettuce Wraps, 74
Chicken Salad with Apricots, 76
Cucumber Roll-Ups, 125
Eggplant Breakfast Sandwich, 48
Game-Day Burger with Jicama Chips, 80–81
Jackfruit Tacos, 103
Miso, Tempeh, and Carrot Wraps, 75
Red Lentil Sloppy Joes with Roasted Asparagus, 78
Roasted Tomato Tartine, 73
Smoked Salmon on Toast, 77
Strawberry-Ricotta Toast, 45
Turkey Pastrami and Pimento Cheese Sandwich, 79
Saturated fats, 20
Sauces
Basic Marinara, 166
Cherry Barbecue Sauce, 165
Peanut Sauce, 168
Romesco Sauce, 170
Sausage, Chicken, and Cauliflower Pizza, 120
Sautéed Lemon Broccoli and Kale, 132
Seedy Muesli, 37
Self-care, 18
Sesame Broccoli, Charred, 135
"Seven Self-Care Behaviors" framework, 18
Shakshuka, 47
Shaved Brussels Sprouts and Kale with Poppy Seed Dressing, 62
Simple Bibimbap, 101
Smashed Cucumber Salad, 136
Smoked Salmon on Toast, 77
Smoked Turkey Chili, 91
Smoothies and shakes
Blueberry-Chia Smoothie, 33
Cherry, Chocolate, and Almond Shake, 34
Snacks
Cucumber Roll-Ups, 125
Eggplant Pizzas, 126
Kale Chip Nachos, 128–129
Lemony White Bean Puree, 130
Roasted Carrot and Chickpea Dip, 127
Sodium, 20
Soups, stews, and chilis
Chickpea Spinach Soup, 88–89
Egg Drop Soup, 83
Golden Chicken Soup, 90
Herbed Buttermilk Chicken, 119
Minted Sweet Pea Soup, 82
Quick Moroccan-Inspired Chicken Stew, 92
Smoked Turkey Chili, 91
Tomato-Basil Soup with Grilled Cheese Croutons, 84–85
West African-Inspired Peanut Soup, 86–87
Spinach
Chickpea Spinach Soup, 88–89
Spinach Salad with Strawberries and Toasted Almonds, 57

Squash, Ribboned, with Bacon, 110
Stovetop Granola, 35–36
Strawberries
  Spinach Salad with Strawberries and Toasted Almonds, 57
  Strawberry-Ricotta Toast, 45
Strawberry-Ricotta Toast, 45
Sugars, 16, 20
Superfood Brownie Bites, 151
Supplements, 10–11
Sweet Beet Grain Bowl, 65
Sweet potatoes, 20
  Kale Chip Nachos, 128–129
  Mashed Sweet Potatoes, 140
  West African–Inspired Peanut Soup, 86–87

# T

Tacos, Jackfruit, 103
Tahini
  Chocolate Tahini Bombs, 155
  Tahini Dressing, 162
  Tahini, Maple, and Banana Overnight Oats, 38
Tempeh, Miso, and Carrot Wraps, 75
Toast
  Smoked Salmon on Toast, 77
  Strawberry-Ricotta Toast, 45
Tofu
  Avocado-Tofu Scramble with Roasted Potatoes, 50–51
  Peanut Tofu over Buckwheat Noodles, 100
Tomatoes
  Basic Marinara, 166
  Cauliflower Steaks with Tomato, Caper, and Golden Raisin Sauce, 104
  Herbed Tomato Salad, 56
  Roasted Asparagus with Romesco Sauce, 133–134
  Roasted Tomato Tartine, 73
  Romesco Sauce, 170
  Shakshuka, 47
  Tomato-Basil Soup with Grilled Cheese Croutons, 84–85
  Tomato, Caper, and Golden Raisin Sauce, 167
  Turkey Bolognese with Chickpea Pasta, 121
Tools, 25–26
Trans fats, 20
Tropical Mango Overnight Oats, 39
Tuna Poke with Riced Broccoli, 105–106
Turkey
  Italian-Style Turkey Meatballs and Zoodles, 109
  Smoked Turkey Chili, 91
  Turkey Bolognese with Chickpea Pasta, 121
  Turkey Pastrami and Pimento Cheese Sandwich, 79
Type 1 diabetes, 5
Type 2 diabetes, 4, 5

# V

Vegetable Mac 'n' Cheese, 102
Vegetarian
  Apple-Bulgur Salad, 64
  Apple Millet Porridge, 40
  Asparagus Salad with Chile-Lime Dressing, 58
  Avocado Slaw, 142
  Avocado-Tofu Scramble with Roasted Potatoes, 50–51
  Banana N'Ice Cream with Cocoa Nuts, 148–149
  Basic Marinara, 166
  Blueberry-Chia Smoothie, 33
  Blueberry Chocolate Clusters, 150
  Breakfast Banana Barley, 41
  Cajun-Style Collards, 139
  Carrot Cake Oatmeal, 44
  Cauliflower Rice, 138

Vegetarian (*continued*)
Cauliflower Steaks with Tomato, Caper, and Golden Raisin Sauce, 104
Cauli-Lettuce Wraps, 74
Charred Miso Cabbage, 141
Charred Sesame Broccoli, 135
Cherry Barbecue Sauce, 165
Cherry, Chocolate, and Almond Shake, 34
Chickpea Fattoush Salad, 67
Chickpea Spinach Soup, 88–89
Chocolate Tahini Bombs, 155
Citrus Avocado Salad, 55
Coconut Macaroons, 154
Cucumber Roll-Ups, 125
Easy Buckwheat Crêpes, 46
Eggplant and Lentils with Curried Yogurt, 98–99
Eggplant Breakfast Sandwich, 48
Eggplant Pizzas, 126
Garlic Roasted Radishes, 137
Gingered Red Lentils with Millet, 97
Grilled Romaine with White Beans, 66
Harissa, 169
Harvest Blackberry Quinoa Bowl, 42
Herbed Tomato Salad, 56
High-Protein Oatmeal, 43
Jackfruit Tacos, 103
Kale Chip Nachos, 128–129
Lemon Vinaigrette Dressing, 159
Lemony White Bean Puree, 130
Mashed Sweet Potatoes, 140
Minted Sweet Pea Soup, 82
Miso, Tempeh, and Carrot Wraps, 75
Orange Praline with Yogurt, 153
Overnight Oats, 38–39
Peanut Sauce, 168
Peanut Tofu over Buckwheat Noodles, 100
Perfect Egg Scramble with Simple Salad, 49
Pickled Carrot and Radish, 172
Pickled Red Onions, 171
Poached Pears, 152
Pomegranate "Tabbouleh" with Cauliflower, 61
Poppy Seed Dressing, 161
Quinoa and Cucumber Salad, 63
Red Lentil Sloppy Joes with Roasted Asparagus, 78
Roasted Asparagus with Romesco Sauce, 133–134
Roasted Carrot and Chickpea Dip, 127
Roasted Carrot and Quinoa with Goat Cheese, 68
Roasted Tomato Tartine, 73
Romesco Sauce, 170
Sautéed Lemon Broccoli and Kale, 132
Seedy Muesli, 37
Shakshuka, 47
Shaved Brussels Sprouts and Kale with Poppy Seed Dressing, 62
Simple Bibimbap, 101
Smashed Cucumber Salad, 136
Spinach Salad with Strawberries and Toasted Almonds, 57
Stovetop Granola, 35–36
Strawberry-Ricotta Toast, 45
Superfood Brownie Bites, 151
Sweet Beet Grain Bowl, 65
Tahini Dressing, 162
Tahini, Maple, and Banana Overnight Oats, 38
Tomato-Basil Soup with Grilled Cheese Croutons, 84–85
Tomato, Caper, and Golden Raisin Sauce, 167

Tropical Mango Overnight Oats, 39
Vegetable Mac 'n' Cheese, 102
Watermelon-Lime Granita, 147
West African–Inspired Peanut Soup, 86–87

## W

Walnut-Crusted Halibut with Pear Salad, 107–108
Watermelon-Lime Granita, 147
West African–Inspired Peanut Soup, 86–87
Whole grains, 20
Wraps. *See* Sandwiches and wraps

## Y

Yams, 20
Yogurt
  Eggplant and Lentils with
    Curried Yogurt, 98–99
  Orange Praline with Yogurt, 153

## Z

Zoodles, Italian-Style Turkey Meatballs and, 109

# Acknowledgments

I would like to thank: My partner Adrian, who inspires me to become a better writer and person, my first chef, JD Fratzke, who taught me how to work the line and cut perfect slices of lardon, the Gallahers, the influential husband-and-wife professor team who taught me to push harder and never stop learning, and all of my friends, family, teachers, and the colleagues who have helped me along the way.

# About the Author

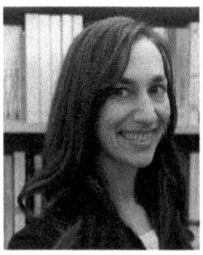

**Ranelle Kirchner, MS, RD, CDCES,** is a licensed registered dietitian, certified diabetic care and education specialist, and Le Cordon Bleu culinary graduate with a passion for health and wellness and a desire to help you understand yours. She runs her own private practice called ChefRDN, LLC, offering nutrition counseling, cooking classes, meal planning, and nutrition education in community and workplace settings. In addition, she is a diabetes educator at Neighborhood Healthsource (NHS), a community nonprofit clinic that brings accessible, affordable care to patients. Learn more by visiting RanelleKirchner.com.